# MUSCULAR
# INDIA

Michiel Baas has a PhD in Anthropology from the University of Amsterdam, and has held various academic positions with the National University of Singapore, Nalanda University (Rajgir), the International Institute for Asian Studies (Leiden) and the University of Amsterdam. Most of his work centres on the Indian middle class. He has published extensively on the topic of fitness and bodybuilding in India; Indian student-migration to Australia; the migration trajectories of skilled professionals in Singapore; the Indian migration industry; and the lives and lifestyles of IT professionals in Bangalore.

I0095682

# Praise for *Muscular India*

'If you are looking for politically correct clichés about masculinity and "changing India", go elsewhere. Enter here for a tender and absorbing story of muscular men, their searching hearts, their quest to matter in the world. In this intricate and often entertaining landscape of gyms and trainers and body building, you glimpse a truth about how vulnerable aspiration makes us, how conditional are the promises of change, and how lonely the enterprise of becoming a man.' – Paromita Vohra, filmmaker, writer and founder, *Agents of Ishq*

'*Muscular India* is an essential addition to the study of upward mobility in India. Through his immersion in the world of gym-made masculinity, Baas brings us unforgettable stories of young men navigating the country's labyrinthine middle class armed with their bodies.' – Snigdha Poonam, author of *Dreamers: How Young Indians Are Changing Their World*

'Baas's rich, textured and deeply insightful ethnography of body building provides us with profoundly important insights on masculinity and sexuality in South Asia. His analysis produces a critically incisive understanding of embodiment, establishing a new and important anthropological perspective on the anxieties and ambivalences of middle-class identity in modern India.' – Joseph S. Alter, author of *The Wrestler's Body: Identity and Ideology in North India* and *Gandhi's Body: Sex, Diet, and the Politics of Nationalism*

'*Muscular India* is a fascinating story of national and bodily transformation, shining a light on the country's rising middle class by way of its muscle men and fitness fanatics. Michiel Baas uses an impressive mix of academic research and colourful real-life "in the gym" stories to reveal a deep urge for self-improvement amongst India's urban elite, from the Bollywood idols whose sculpted bodies they emulate to the ambitious working-class men who train and encourage them.' – James Crabtree, author of *The Billionaire Raj: A Journey through India's New Gilded Age*

'Michiel Baas uses bodybuilding and the gym culture to provide deep insights into the Indian middle class, notions of mobility, cultures of consumption, the obsession with Bollywood bodies and sexual desire. Based on years of ethnographic research, the book is invaluable in understanding the paradoxes of urban India.' – Ronojoy Sen, author of *Nation at Play: A History of Sport in India*

'What do body building and the muscular body mean in contemporary India? To this apparently straightforward question, Michiel Baas provides a series of fascinating answers that capture the extraordinary social and cultural churn in contemporary Indian society. An academic readership will discover new ways of thinking of the body as an exploration of social life whereas a non-academic one will discover what accessible scholarly analysis has to offer towards a nuanced understanding of the Indian present.' – Sanjay Srivastava, author of *Entangled Urbanism: Slum, Gated Community and Shopping Mall in Delhi and Gurgaon*

'It's rare to find a study that effectively combines theory and practice, but Michiel Baas's study of masculinity and the middle class in India does just that. *Muscular India* is conceptually sophisticated and ethnographically immersive; it moves fluently from idea to detail, and back, all the while introducing us to a cast of well-rounded characters who play out their lives in fascinating, little-explored settings. Along the way, the book also makes detours into a host of important contemporary issues, including consumerism, urbanisation, sexual mores, food adulteration and the nation's technology industry. What all of this adds up to is a nuanced and layered portrait of modern India.' – Akash Kapur, author of *India Becoming: A Portrait of Life in Modern India*

'Through his illustrative and eloquent writing, Michiel Baas takes us on a vivid journey through the bumpy, aspirational worlds of lower-middle-class male fitness trainers in India. In all its ethnographic vitality, the author successfully captures how a poignant search for economic status and social respectability intersects with the desire for muscularity and transformed bodies among these men. Baas's lucid and nuanced reflections, on how these robustly modelled bodies become emblematic of a new India, is a must-read for those interested in the expanding market for body-building in middle-class and urban India.' – Atreyee Sen, author of *Shiv Sena Women: Violence and Communalism in a Bombay Slum*

'Baas's study is nuanced—he steers clear of generalisations, letting his subjects speak for themselves. The book's experiential quality gives it authenticity besides making it eminently readable.' – *The Hindu*

'In tracing one of the less noticed, and far less examined, strands of mobility within middle-class India, and its constraints, *Muscular India* is an important contribution to the understanding of urban India. As a project of self-fashioning, to borrow a historian's description, still explains the nature of the Indian middle class, the book shows new ways of looking at the new entrants and the influential gatekeepers of this project in urban India.' – *Newslaundry*

# MUSCULAR
## INDIA
### MASCULINITY, MOBILITY
### AND THE NEW MIDDLE CLASS

## MICHIEL BAAS

# cntxt

First published in hardback by Context, an imprint of Westland Publications Private Limited, in 2020

First published in paperback by Context, an imprint of Westland Books, a division of Nasadiya Technologies Private Limited, in 2022

No. 269/2B, First Floor, 'Irai Arul', Vimalraj Street, Nethaji Nagar, Allappakkam Main Road, Maduravoyal, Chennai 600095

Westland, the Westland logo, Context and the Context logo are the trademarks of Nasadiya Technologies Private Limited, or its affiliates.

Copyright © Michiel Baas, 2020

Michiel Baas asserts the moral right to be identified as the author of this work.

ISBN: 9789395073622

10 9 8 7 6 5 4 3 2 1

The views and opinions expressed in this work are the author's own and the facts are as reported by him, and the publisher is in no way liable for the same.

All rights reserved

Typeset by SÜRYA, New Delhi

Printed at Parksons Graphics Pvt Ltd

No part of this book may be reproduced, or stored in a retrieval system, or transmitted in any form or by any means, electronic, mechanical, photocopying, recording, or otherwise, without express written permission of the publisher.

*For Rithesh*

# CONTENTS

# INTRODUCTION

It took three movies and a magazine to popularise a new bodily ideal among middle-class men in India, characterised by bulging biceps, rock-hard abs and visibly pronounced pecs. Radiating masculine strength and athleticism, this ideal diverges markedly from the healthy potbelly of yesteryear's middle-class male—once the signifier of prosperity and well-being. This new ideal does not align easily with that of the pehlwan-wrestler whose body is the product of a diet rich in ghee, almonds and cow milk. Even if there is some tangible (or historical) connection in terms of workout routines, the end result is a radically different body. While this new lean and muscular body, with its emphasis on vascularity, comes closer to that of the working classes, within a middle-class context it now references discipline, professionalism and cosmopolitanism. While this trend has been taking shape for roughly two decades, it's only in the last ten years or so that it has caused a veritable fitness boom across India.

For an older generation of fitness trainers and bodybuilders, Salman Khan's hit-movie *Pyaar Kiya to Darna Kya* (1998) was the first intimation of what could be achieved with their bodies. However, this only translated into the real and very rapid growth in gym memberships and demand for personal training when Shah Rukh Khan revealed his freshly baked six-pack abs in *Om Shanti Om* (2007). The actor's dramatic transformation was a hot topic of discussion in popular media that year. Yet, this was nothing compared to what would befall Aamir Khan after he starred in *Ghajini* (2008), the Hindi remake of a 2005 Tamil blockbuster, itself based on the American *Memento* (2000).[1] Shot not long after he played an art teacher and 'ordinary' boy-next-door in *Taare Zameen Par* (2007), in *Ghajini* the actor sports a phenomenally muscular physique that immediately begged the question: how had he pulled it off? In 2007, the Indian edition of *Men's Health* was launched, further propelling the creed of the lean, muscular body. The magazine's use of cover models who were not celebrities confirmed the potential of the Indian male body beyond Bollywood's elite.

What is this body about, though? Why has it so seized the imagination of middle-class men? And where have these legions of fitness and personal trainers emerged from? After a decade spent researching this phenomenon, I believe that the notion of transformation is key to understanding these developments. Bollywood actors constantly discuss the details of how they have sculpted their body to specifically suit a new movie project, making it part of promotional activities. In fact, this bodily transformation is often a separate storyline in itself, to be narrated alongside that of the movie in question. It draws attention to the lead actor's body as something to go see and admire in addition to the movie's actual storyline. Gyms too aggressively promote the potential for transformation, often imbuing it with notions that venture well beyond the idea of fitness per se. *Men's Health* magazine even suggested that transforming one's body wasn't merely about health and fitness but also about being professional, cosmopolitan and 'in control' to withstand the caprices of rampant overconsumption.

Meanwhile, there is no denying that India itself is transforming. Cities are rapidly expanding, new places of leisure and consumption open their doors all the time, and quality of life—due to air pollution, population growth and the pressure on existing infrastructure—is diminishing. Central to these developments is the growth of the middle class itself. While it tends to be the middle class that cities cater to as they expand, remake and introduce new ways of consumption and leisure, it also presents them with new opportunities in terms of career pathways and generating an income.

This book builds upon an almost decade-long research engagement with lower-middle-class men for whose families the very idea of belonging to the Indian middle class is a relatively new situation. Employed as fitness (or personal) trainers and competing in bodybuilding and modelling competitions, these men's muscular bodies appear to reflect the very promise of a new India. Through extensive physical transformation, their bodies have come to approximate the lean and muscular ideal that Bollywood has popularised. The last decade or so has seen the rapid emergence of a fitness industry across India, attracting an ever-growing number of middle-class Indians struggling with issues of weight-gain and aspiring to achieve this new muscular ideal. Trainers and bodybuilders have become brokers in bodily knowledge and are held to have the key to physical transformation. As much as they are admired for their bodies, the socio-economic distance between the trainers—hailing from lower-middle-class vernacular ('vernac') backgrounds—and their clients remains significant. However, this ostensive class gap also presents an opportunity for social mobility.

Interacting with upper-middle-class clients helps trainers improve their English and acquire knowledge of the kind of lifestyles they aspire to. Their bodies function almost literally as currency in this; it buys them a way into something that would have otherwise kept its doors resolutely shut. At the same time, these relationships between trainers and clients continue to be revealing for the boundaries that separate different layers of the Indian middle class, pointing at the resilience of entrenched hierarchies. As much as change and limitless opportunities characterise the narrative of a new and rapidly changing India, upward socioeconomic mobility can be a pretty sluggish process as well.

## A New and Changing 'Middle-Class' India

For decades now, the dominant narrative about India is of a country undergoing rapid change, and emerging as an economic and geopolitical force to be reckoned with. This idea of a *changing* or *new* India can be traced back to the year 1997, when the country celebrated the fiftieth anniversary of its Independence. Around this theme of a half-century-year-old nation, international media focused on the concept of transformation and the country's growing dominance in the world of information technology. Popular magazines with an international readership, such as *Business Week*, *The Economist*, *Newsweek* and *Time*, often drew upon the dyad of the elephant and the tiger or a variety thereof. The former symbolised an India of the past, shackled by a planned economy and Licence Raj, something that came to an end in 1991 when the country's economy was liberalised and foreign capital started flowing in. In contrast, post-1991, India was increasingly equated with a tiger, roaring loudly and ready to show the world its teeth. These analyses and stories neatly juxtaposed *old* (black-and-white) images of the political leaders who had ushered in Independence and the years of despair that followed with *new*, colourful ones of IT campuses, shopping malls and the flamboyancy of Bollywood. Central to these developments appeared to be the emerging Indian middle class with its command of the English language, transnationally marketable skills and new consumer power. In the years that followed, the question of what precisely this change entailed beyond these generalisations resulted in a number of studies and essays, often with a specific focus on the Indian middle class. *Muscular India* takes inspiration from these but is also critical of them.

Even those studies that do acknowledge that middle-class India is not a homogenous whole, rarely is there an examination of how the various layers that characterise the middle class relate to each other, or how more recent members of the middle class may strategise to close the gap with those considered higher or 'upper'. Instead, the middle class's internal hierarchy—characterised by a (newer, vernacular) lower middle class and (older, English-speaking upper middle class)—is often somewhat unwittingly reproduced. The chapters to come challenge this in that they focus on those whose ambition it is to climb the middle-class ladder. Even before Indian Independence, new entrants were perceived as 'inauthentic' and inherently suspect, equated with materialism and other types of behaviour frowned upon by the old elite. Born out of a lack of capable (British) administrative staff who could keep the colonial engine going, the formation of an older middle class can be traced to Lord T.B. Macaulay's 1835 'Minute on Indian Education', which suggested that: 'We must at present do our best to form a class who may be interpreters between us and the millions we govern; a class of persons, Indian in blood and colour, but English in taste, in opinions, in morals, and in intellect.'[2] Even if this class later came to frown upon new entrants, during colonial times, they themselves were perceived to be 'deracinated hybrids who could never hope to be fully Western, and who, at the same time, were cut off from their own culture and civilization because of their exposure to Western ideas'.[3] In this regard, the emerging middle class of colonial India compared unfavourably with an allegedly more authentic one that had its roots in Europe and the US.[4]

In his perceptive study of the making of a colonial middle class in north India, historian Sanjay Joshi (2001) notes how 'being middle class' was mainly a project of self-fashioning. His assertion that the middle class needs to be understood as a project that was constantly in the making and not simply as a mere sociological fact is something that continues to hold relevance for new middle-class formation in contemporary India. To be modern in colonial India meant centring the notion of aspiration,[5] which is also how India's new middle class is conceptualised.

Well-known author Pavan K. Varma, who was one of the first to address the question of the Indian middle class in his appropriately titled *The Great Indian Middle Class* (1999), voiced his concern about the new middle class's proclivity to uncritically copy everything that comes from the West.[6] In a somewhat similar vein, sociologist and public intellectual Dipankar Gupta phrased his unease through the notion of westoxification.[7] In the slipstream of such studies, a more transnational perspective on the formation of middle-class identities and lifestyles emerged as well. In these we find that middle-class avariciousness and apathy is fuelled by the growing gap between a globally connected, transnationally oriented middle class and those left behind in this growth model. Geographer Emma Mawdsley (2004) writes that members of this globally connected middle class appear to have more in common with other middle classes in countries such as Australia, South Africa and the US than with what she describes as the 'parochialised "have-nots" of their own nation.'[8]

## Three Hundred Million Middle-Class Indians

On 3 February 2014, the cover of *Open* magazine featured a drawing of a fictive scene bringing together the two competing electoral prime-ministerial candidates at the time, Narendra Modi (Bharatiya Janata Party, BJP) and Rahul Gandhi (Congress). Sitting on a wooden bench facing a calm river, both have their fishing rods out, about to haul in the middle-class vote. 'The baiting of the middle class' is how *Open* captures the issue at hand. 'This 300 million strong constituency is now clamouring for political attention—and getting it too.'[9] Accompanying the article is an illustration of both political leaders in a boat, this time decidedly less composed, standing up, fishing lines ramrod straight, and bewitched masses emerging from the murky-blue waters below, having caught the bait.[10] The focus of the piece is resolutely on the *new* middle class, which according to well-known academic Ashis Nandy had 'emerged as a formidable force in the country' [and who now] 'constitute more than one-fourth of the population.'[11] The middle class would indeed play a key role in the 2014 elections in which Narendra Modi secured a landslide victory. Five years later, the mandate from the middle class appears to only have increased. While, in 2004, the BJP's use of the slogan 'India Shining' backfired and is held to have contributed to the defeat of then prime minister Atal Bihari Vajpayee's BJP-led government, ten years later the promise of a new and shining India was very much integral to the construction of 'Brand Modi', with its emphasis on the successes made in his home state (Gujarat), the fight he pledged against corruption, and his appeal to urban voters and India's youth.[12] Even though Modi rarely directly referred to the promise of a new and shining India during the 2014 campaign, the victory speeches he made right afterwards explicitly did.[13] Having successfully hauled in the 300-million-strong middle-class vote, a new India was (again) ready to take off.

How do new middle-class Indians relate to the idea of change and the opportunities it brings? While studies of the Indian middle class tend to take economic growth as a point of departure to discuss the rapid emergence of a new class of consumers with significant political influence, their estimations of size are revealing. For one, the number of 300 million has existed for at least two decades now. In *India: Globalization and Change* (2000), anthropologist Pamela Shurmer-Smith already speaks of 300 million, drawing on data from the late 1990s. Even though she herself appeared unconvinced that this was correct at the time, it is clear that it concerned an estimate that had had some traction for a while already.[14] In contrast, the *Far Eastern Economic Review* (FEER) estimated the middle class as just over a 100 million or 12 per cent of the total population in 1993.[15] Even if India's economic liberalisations were only two years old at the time, surely the middle class didn't grow by 200 million individuals over the next seven years? Confusingly, six years after Shurmer-Smith's book was published, anthropologist Minna Säävälä (2006) speaks of 200 million, or 20 per cent of India's population, in her study of new middle-class aspirations in Hyderabad. Säävälä borrows this figure from sociologist D.L. Sheth's study which appeared in 1999, only one year before Shurmer-Smith's.[16] In contrast, political scientist Leela Fernandes's influential publication *India's New Middle Classes* (2006), which appeared in the same year as Säävälä's, speaks of a 250 million-strong middle-class consumer market.[17]

More recent studies continue to befuddle. In their introduction to the edited volume *Elite and Everyman*, Amita Baviskar and Raka Ray (2011) write that '[w]ith the broadest definition of the middle class in India, it is estimated that the top 26 per cent of Indian households belong to this income group.'[18] For this they refer to E. Sridharan's work (2004)[19], which focuses on dissecting the sectorial composition of the country's middle classes but whose data set does not go beyond the year 2000. In a widely quoted publication of 2004 (reprinted in the earlier mentioned 2011 volume), E. Sridharan himself acknowledges the maddening diversity in terms of size estimates, saying it varies between 50, 150 million and 250 million. In her detailed and insightful study of middle-class anxieties and gender in Madurai (Tamil Nadu), Sara Dickey (2012) notes that estimations of the size of India's middle classes vary between 50 and 350 million, corresponding with at least 5 per cent and at most 35 per cent of India's population.[20] However, Dickey also adds that there is growing agreement that the higher figures are greatly exaggerated.[21] Surinder S. Jodhka and Aseem Prakash note something similar in their book in the Oxford India Short Introductions, *The Indian Middle Class* (2016), arguing that estimates vary between 'a lower end of 5 or 6 per cent of the total population' and 'an upper end of 25 or 30 per cent, and sometimes, even more.'[22]

## A (Negative) Product of Economic Growth

Discussions about size also point to highly specific ways of thinking about what the middle class stands for. There is a tendency to focus primarily on consumption and political influence.[23] The article in *Open* suggests that the two are directly related—by making 'their' size count, India's middle class is all about consumerism and demanding politics to cater to their needs. This resonates with a popular framing of the new middle class as chiefly unethical, narcissistic and uninterested in the larger issues India grapples with, be it poverty, environmental pollution or violence against minorities. The adjective 'new', therefore, does not so much refer to an expanding middle class in positive terms—denoting upward socioeconomic mobility— but rather a ballooning one, not unlike a protruding waistline. The new middle class is not celebrated as an outcome of economic growth but seen as a negative by-product instead, signifying a society out of control.

However, as sensitive and ethnographically rich studies such as Ritty A. Lukkose's *Liberalization's Children* (2009), Christiane Brosius's *India's Middle Class* (2010) and Sara Dickey's *Living Class in Urban India* (2012) confirm, the idea of a singular 'united' middle class with a clear consumerist and political agenda is deeply problematic. Instead, what stands out is how complex the middle class's internal hierarchical layering and regional differences can be. *Muscular India* uses the term 'middle class' to mean a purely social and cultural construct. The use of lower, middle and upper middle class in everyday-speak does not only indicate economic difference but also points at an interplay of other factors. Fitness trainers and bodybuilders tend to hail from working class or lower-middle-class backgrounds. Using the appeal of their muscular physiques and their knowledge of how bodies can transform to achieve that effect, these men (it is an overwhelmingly male field) generate an income out of the bodily aspiration of their upper-middle-class clients. In doing so, they also capitalise on what clients perceive these muscular bodies to stand for. Yet, the muscular body alone cannot compensate for the socioeconomic gap that characterises the relationship that clients have with their trainers. Climbing the middle-class ladder, making alternative career decisions, or simply doing things differently, requires long-term investments in generating social and cultural capital. The new middle-class profession of providing fitness training offers a unique opportunity for this since it requires a long-term, and often deeply personal, commitment between trainer and client. At the same time, trainer–client relations continue to be illuminating for the boundaries and obstacles that lower-middle-class men face when strategising toward upward socioeconomic and cultural mobility.

## New Middle-Class Professionals

The profession of fitness or personal trainer, much like that of coffee barista and shop attendant in high-end malls, has emerged out of economic growth itself. These professions are characterised by new ways of working, often requiring direct contact with clients and customers. At Starbucks, for instance, this revolves around the idea of creating a 'third space' for customers—an alternative to the home or office space. Baristas are specifically encouraged to make customers feel at home by engaging in chitchat, inquiring about their day and learning their names and preferences, something unheard of in the fast-food outlets and eateries they may have otherwise found employment at.[24] In the case of providing fitness training, this contact tends to go much deeper. Besides, trainers are the physical manifestation of something their clients desire, something that money cannot necessarily buy: a muscular body characterised by bulging biceps, clearly pronounced pecs and rock-hard abs. However, those successful in the field of fitness training are rarely able to rely on their bodies alone. They must be able to successfully interact with clients as well as translate the customer's vision into training routines and dietary regimes. A certain middle-class comportment is deemed crucial to this, something that could even be understood as being sufficiently able to perform middle-class belonging.

These professions are relatively new, and the trainers are self-made men, not just in terms of having fashioned and precision-engineered their bodies, but also having developed a career or business trajectory out of this involvement. Parents and other family members are generally far from supportive of these trajectories, and their personal histories are revealing for how so many have taken considerable financial risks. Largely educated in a 'vernacular' language, instead of the 'English-medium' that characterises their clients' upper-middle-class upbringing, these men are up against another hurdle to overcome. Bodily capital, as such, is rarely enough to compensate for a lack of social and cultural capital, and can even complicate matters. The trainers whose ambition it is to rise in bodybuilding ranks through locally, regionally and (inter)nationally held competitions have to work towards a muscular body that might deviate from the ideal-type that their upper-middle-class clients are after. It might even render them 'too large' for mainstream gyms who are keen to avoid the (older) association of such bodies with underworld or goonda characters. So, trainers must find a balance where their body might still appeal even if it is not something the client ambitions for himself. And this is crucial: the muscular ideal is never quite stable and not every muscular body appeals to the middle-class imagination. Trainers interviewed who worked with Bollywood (Hindi), Kollywood (Tamil) and Sandalwood (Kannadiga) stars all confirmed that, increasingly, actors start with the question of what type of muscular body they want to display in their next movie. An actor will be able to capitalise on the body he presents through the narrative of transformation, even if the end result is not necessarily one that fitness enthusiasts might want to emulate.

## Sizing Up the Middle Class

It is striking how central questions of size are to discussions about the Indian middle class as well as the ideal and appeal of the muscular body. When I brought this up over drinks with a friend in Delhi, he humorously suggested that 'of course size matters!' While he was not necessarily referring to the middle class itself, his rambunctious involvement in regularly held gay parties across the city spoke of a certain middle-class belonging where opportunities for same-sex encounters were in abundance. As an English-educated and highly paid professional working for a multinational company, my friend clearly belonged to a different bracket of society than some of the trainers he had allegedly seduced in his gym's steam room. Even if such men did not identify as gay themselves, my friend assumed that their 'vernacular' backgrounds meant that these encounters signified something entirely different for them than they did for himself. It aligned with a sort of general perception among clients that trainers would be at their every beck and call, providing them with dietary advice, lifestyle tips and providing exceptional flexibility in terms of their personal training schedules. The understanding was that 'these men' might be open to same-sex encounters due to the more conservative (traditional) gender relations in their communities, which greatly reduced the chance of casual sexual relations with members of the opposite sex. There was also, of course, the assumption that the trainers' socioeconomic backgrounds leave them with no choice but to be available, flexible and 'servile'. It sketches a divide between 'opposing' middle-class camps that would often percolate through casual banter; something I have come to be intensely critical of. As much as upper-middle-class opinions of lower-middle-class newcomers were built on an intrinsic dyad (vernacular vs English; provincial vs cosmopolitan; boorish vs cultured), interactions and relations between the two were revealing for how little is truly set in stone.

A pertinent question about the Indian middle class is precisely what its potential represents. In other words, what can be found between India's increasingly muscular legs? This is a question that arises from the fact that much of the discussion about the Indian middle class, as well as the country's economic growth and its swelling geopolitical influence, abounds in masculine overtones. Mother India and her association with Gandhi's struggle for Independence and Nehru's post-1947 planned-economy period, has gradually been replaced with the notion of a boisterous awakening, a sleeping giant getting on its feet, and a country showing its might to the world. As noted earlier, this narrative is replete with the flexing of muscles. Inescapable here is the liberalisation of India's economy in 1991, in which the gradual abolition of the licence-raj was a crucial element. During this phase, domestic capital was freed from licensing constraints, import restrictions were reduced, the currency devalued, and opportunities for Foreign Direct Investment increased. As a result, it became much easier and more appealing to invest in India, which in turn encouraged a rapidly growing number of multinationals to establish offices in India.[25]

More recently, the country's twenty-fifth anniversary of economic liberalisations has led to revisiting the 1991 period and, in particular, to a renewed assessment of its much-maligned prime minister of the time, P.V. Narasimha Rao.[26] While the reforms that were implemented followed a succession of severe financial crises, this history now also functions as a pivotal moment: that's when new India took off. Yet the exuberance that clings to this narrative is also somewhat duplicitous because it ignores genuine questions about the number of Indians who have actually benefited from economic developments since.

## UPGRADING MIDDLE-CLASSNESS

Besides an important new way of generating an income, the fitness training industry also represents an opportunity to 'do things differently'. Not following in their father's footsteps, nor joining the family business, or opting for a 'respectable' salaried job, such as engineering, medicine or accounting, the trainers that this book focuses on are part of a growing group of young Indians who attempt to carve out a non-traditional career trajectory. Part of the industry's attraction is that it is seen as an *opportunity to learn*, which ranges from improving one's English language to learning new business and networking skills. Working in high-end gyms allows trainers to develop a deeper understanding of the lives and lifestyles of their upper-middle-class clients, something they hope will be handy in 'upgrading' their own lives. The term 'upgrading'—frequently employed to describe the work on their own bodies—was also used to define their ambitions beyond the gym. I hung out regularly in a small neighbourhood gym in South Delhi (see chapter two), which was deeply informative for how trainers give shape and direction to such ambitions. It was equally revealing for how their upper-middle-class clients perceived and engaged with these attempts at upward mobility.

Supriya,[27] one of the female clients at this gym, well aware of my research, would often probe me for updates about my progress. Most mornings she was trained by Amit, a floor trainer who took a selection of regulars under his wing and provided them with on-the-spot instructions on what exercises to do next. Amit was originally from Chirag Dilli, another South Delhi neighbourhood, though of a decidedly different standing from CR Park or GK-1,[28] where most of the gym's clients hailed from. In fact, Chirag Dilli is officially designated as an 'urban village'.[29] Each day early morning, Amit made his way from this 'village' to GK in order to provide the gym's clients with personal guidance. Although he had received almost all of his education in Hindi, he was always keen to speak English inside the gym as a way of practising the language, which he considered crucial to his future success as a personal trainer. For this reason, Supriya had also taken him under her wing and often rather adamantly insisted on speaking English, something she herself was fluent in due to her upper-middle-class upbringing.[30] This native Hindi and Punjabi speaker spoke in an English laced with words and sentences in Hindi for purposes of clarification as well as the freedom it provided to mock Amit in a jovial manner.

One morning, Supriya asked, waving her hand casually in Amit's direction, 'What is it precisely that you want to know about them?' I explained that I was mainly approaching the topic from the angle of it representing a new middle-class profession that does not only offer alternative career prospects but also opportunities for upward social mobility. 'For instance, because of their almost daily interaction with people like you here in the gym.' Supriya remained silent for a while and then offered me her opinion: 'I see what you are saying, it is indeed remarkable how good these guys are at mimicking middle-class behaviour.' Her use of the word 'mimicking' indicated that she certainly did not consider Amit her equal. In fact, she seemed to doubt that such a thing was even possible. She smiled and added: 'They try really hard you know.' She had observed herself how trainers like Amit were 'practising middle-classness' through their interactions with her and other clients. Even as she tried to help Amit out with his English, she continued to play the part of gatekeeper, someone who decides what is sufficiently middle class. In a nutshell, this is what most trainers of new middle-class backgrounds struggle with. Understanding the language, codes and norms of middle-class belonging took time and effort. This slow-paced process contrasted with how fast everything else seemed to be developing.

## Awareness of the Ostensive Gap

As new middle-class professionals, the fitness trainers in this book have embarked on a career trajectory that none of their family members have experience in. Parents tend to have very limited understanding of what this work entails, and trainers often struggle to convince the family that their work is of a genuine nature and not connected to underworld or goonda practices. More generally, this also means a new way of thinking about themselves in relation to their immediate environment and India's changing urban landscape. As new entrants to the middle class, these men are part of a growing group of Indians who are actively testing the flexibility of, and manoeuvrability within, Indian society. However, while celebrating the opportunities this brings in terms of breaking through class boundaries and facilitating socioeconomic mobility, it is not hard to see how fitness companies themselves understand this and seek to profit from these young men's ambitions. A manager of Gold's Gym (a franchise operation of American origin) in the north of Delhi was very clear that he expected his team to 'build a rapport with their customers so that they can cash [in] on that'. His objectives were simple: 'I want sales!' He would tell his trainers exactly how to communicate with their clients. He described it as wanting them to do this 'in a slightly higher way'. What he meant by this, he clarified, was the unlearning of some of their ways of speaking—'in a rough, lower-class way'—and 'to add some maturity' to the way they conducted themselves. His battalion of trainers, who were neatly lined up in his office during the interview, were not to only think of the members as clients to be made money of but also ensure they were genuinely comfortable coming to the gym. Most of his trainers were of Gujjar[31] and Jat backgrounds, and their brusque nature might upset the well-heeled clients of the gym, the manager suggested (see also chapter five). What stands out is how aware he was of the gap that existed between his clientele and staff. He saw himself as an interlocutor here, somebody who firmly understood the gym's predicament: catering to upper-middle-class clients while relying on lower-middle-class trainers.

This gap in middle-classness is not just characterised by socioeconomic distance but also what could be seen as a space of mobility. Both tangible and intangible forms of mobility play a role. On the one hand, there is the highly concrete notion of upward economic mobility, which is usually treated as one that can be proven with statistics. It is not hard to see how upward economic mobility resonates and runs parallel to advances in physical mobility: acquiring a motorcycle, the transition to a first car, and the upward trajectory in terms of brands—from Nano to Indigo to Jaguar.[32] This contrasts with the evanescent and slippery nature of social and cultural mobility. Economic mobility almost always runs parallel to processes of upward social mobility (expanding one's network, gradually inhabiting a different social layer of society altogether) and sideward cultural mobility (doing things differently, exploring alternative pathways). Treating these different forms of mobility— economic, physical, social and cultural—as essentially conflated, part and parcel of the same trajectory helps develop a much deeper perspective of the way newness and change comes about in India.

## Intersecting Mobilities and Intangible Forms of Capital

Research in the field of social mobility tends to be of an objectivist nature, often taking a quantitative and decidedly aggregated approach.[33] John Goldthorpe's social mobility studies that were conducted from the mid-1970s onward set the initial tone for the field. His team's methods left little space for the role of ambivalence, missteps and side-trajectories.[34] Pierre Bourdieu (1987) spoke of the biographical illusion here, pointing at the fallacy of coherence and meaning projected onto an individual's life narrative. An additional problem is that previous studies were rarely situated in a context of rapid change, such as is the case in India. Instead, they tend to employ a long-term, even cross-generational, focus that differs considerably from the one utilised throughout this book. As such, the Indian context necessitates a deviation or rethinking from the classical understanding of what social and cultural mobility entails. In the Bourdieuan sense, social capital dwells in and is produced through social relations, memberships of the right clubs, and 'simply' via interaction with others. These relations or connections are more than just that; the key is knowing how to capitalise on them.[35] Social mobility's innately slippery nature comes to the fore when we realise that it is often a by-product of activities engaged in for other purposes.[36] There is something self-evident or self-fulfilling about social mobility that goes to the heart of the very nature of social capital. It reproduces in a progressively cumulative manner; social capital produces social capital and then some. Ronald Stuart Burt (2000) pointed out that those who do better in life are generally also better connected. Those born in the right families tend to have better connections, (hereditary) memberships in the right clubs and organisations—think of the Bangalore Club, Delhi's India International Centre, or the Madras Club in Chennai—and in all likelihood will enrol in better schools, colleges and universities. The advantage here is not only the network one is born into but also the lifelong opportunity one has to understand how this network works and make use of its membership.

Cultural capital—unlike social capital, which functions beneath the surface—more obviously allocates a particular intangible value to a person. Studies show education as particularly instrumental in contributing to this, even if it has also been considered for its potential as the great equaliser—lifting people out of poverty and closing the gap between rich and poor. As Craig Jeffrey's (2010) pathbreaking work focusing on the context of provincial (tier two) India has shown, education alone rarely has all the answers. While young men in India's smaller towns have increasingly become more educated because of reservation policies and state-led investments in higher education, this has not necessarily translated into better opportunities. Pierre Bourdieu (1986) distinguished various forms of cultural capital (embodied, objectified and institutionalised) that helps sort out the complexity we see. There is the embodied state of cultural capital: cultural capital is most of all something one strategically reveals or makes visible, to which a certain degree of effortlessness would be key. In other words, what could be understood as middle-class comportment. I once introduced long-term informant and trainer Kishore to a friend who hailed from an upper-middle-class background, and who was interested in including him in a documentary-film project. My friend observed how Kishore had made such an effort 'to look the part'. It reminded me of what Supriya had said about mimicking middle-class behaviour. For it to be convincing, it has to appear natural, which is a strain for most trainers since their family's membership to the middle class is a relatively recent development. Unable to draw upon 'intimate' internalised knowledge of how to blend in effortlessly, the danger is that it might look too studied. This touches upon the physical (objectified) or visible dimension of cultural capital. In a Western context, this is symbolised by (the ownership of) books, dictionaries and instruments. However, in the case of India, it is not unreasonable to expand this to clothes and other objects, such as cars and mobile phones, that may not strictly embody knowledge but that are held to 'represent' a particular 'knowing' of what they stand for in a middle-class context. Kishore, for one, no longer buys his 'branded' clothes from the local bazaar, instead investing in the 'real thing' because his clients would immediately pick up on them being counterfeit. These much more expensive clothes are not only meant to underline that he knows what appeals to his clients, but also that he understands the socioeconomic stratum they inhabit (and which he ambitions to become part of himself). The institutionalised state of cultural capital, represented by educational qualifications, complements and further strengthens this.[37] In India, education remains one of the main qualifiers of middle-class belonging. However, it is not only the reputation of the institution that matters, but equally if not more so, the language of education. The very idea of 'vernacular'—as in education, upbringing, mode of communication (at home, with friends)—has even taken on the character of a swear word, as evidenced by its use in the Amazon hit-show *Made in Heaven*, which revolves around two wedding planners in Delhi. Jazz, one of the assistants who is originally from Dwarka (a sub-city and diplomatic enclave in Southwest Delhi), tries to make it in the far more posh and opulent setting of South Delhi. When she is unable to meet the wishes of one of the agency's wealthy clients, she is called a 'bloody vernac'.[38]

Social and cultural capital come together in Bourdieu's (1990) use of the concept of 'habitus', which speaks of a system of dispositions through which we perceive, judge and act in the world. It ensures the active presence (and influence) of past experiences, embodied and internationalised so it is second nature.[39] Even the way we bear our bodies could almost immediately give away our place in society. We appear to ooze this habitus through our pores; like pheromones, it is something others pick up on without necessarily realising it. Famously, Edward Palmer Thompson once described the habitus as a 'feel for the game'.[40] While this book doesn't speak of a middle-class habitus—as its set-in-stone character doesn't necessarily easily translate to the rapidly changing Indian urban context—it is in essence what *Muscular India* seeks to investigate. What does it take to become middle class? Or perhaps more succinctly: what does it take to convincingly pull off the idea of 'confidently' belonging to the middle class? As a new entrant, how does one lose the skin of newness, one's entry being suspect and up for inspection and judgement? Even if this requires navigating the treacherous pathway from lower to upper middle class, the eventual end goal is not to become 'like them', but to take up a space of one's own. In that sense, what we witness here is a much longer-term continuation of new middle-class formation where notions of new/lower and older/upper have always been in motion and flux. As a social and cultural construct, middle-class belonging, no matter one's socioeconomic standing, is always criticised, suspicious and in question.

# CHAPTER 1

# THE NEW INDIAN MALE

*'We are kings of this world, man!'*

– Vijay, personal trainer

Kishore's muscles glisten in the hot afternoon sun as he speeds towards me on his customised shiny-black Royal Enfield motorcycle, bare-chested and waving enthusiastically. If this were a Bollywood movie, the soundtrack's incessant and asynchronous drumming would have coalesced into one coherent rhythm by now, followed by Kishore stepping off his motorcycle, tossing his Ray-Ban aviators into a crowd of swooning onlookers and commencing his dance routine. His neatly torn Levi's and sturdy boots would complement the scene.

Yet, the street is oddly empty, and even the Hanuman temple where he asked me to wait seems quiet for the time of day. He beckons me to jump onto the back of his bike and we drive off towards Chembur, a working-class neighbourhood of Mumbai, where he grew up. The celebrations for the final day of Ganesh Chaturthi are in full swing.[41] In his usual animated fashion, Kishore summarises the past few days of the festival while deftly navigating traffic. He ploughs through groups of energetically dancing men moving to the sound of dhols. All of them are readying for the long journey to the seashore, where murtis[42] of the elephant god will be immersed in the water. I had encountered countless such street parties over the past few days. Mumbai had come to a relative standstill, with businesses shuttered, streets closed to traffic and throngs of crowds queuing until late into the night to receive a coveted blessing at one of the makeshift pandals[43] where local communities instal their towering Ganesha idols. For ten to eleven days each year, Mumbai—India's financial heart—dances not to the tune of money, but to the percussive rhythm of the worship of its beloved patron deity.

The fourteen-foot-tall Ganesha seems to loom over Khardev Nagar in Chembur where people from Kishore's neighbourhood have gathered to celebrate. A chaotic party has started in front of the cart on which the murti is mounted. The air is thick with the smell of incense and sweat, and Bollywood music blasts from speakers even as drummers compete deliriously for attention. When we get closer, we notice Vijay, who is taking off his T-shirt and tucking it into his belt while a crowd of onlookers observes his every move. As lean and muscular as Kishore, his body is the product of martial arts, boxing and functional training. Both in their late twenties, their similarities in physique and style continue to their sunglasses and nearly identical motorcycles, which Kishore now indicates we will take for a spin around Chembur to inspect some of the other pandals. We might even be able to buy some liquor on the way, Vijay suggests, despite it being a dry day.[44]

As we cruise around Chembur, we're regularly pulled over by Kishore and Vijay's friends and acquaintances who want to know where we're heading, and to admire their physiques. There is no denying the spectacle on offer: sculpted muscles, perfectly V-shaped backs, protruding calves and upper-legs, and biceps that flex with every animated gesture. They happily pose with bystanders for pictures hurriedly taken with mobile phones and then analysed. Fingers zoom in on particular muscle groups, followed by keen inquiries about workout tips and diet suggestions. Jokes are made referencing Bollywood stars Hrithik Roshan and Salman Khan, to whom this duo is considered to have a vague resemblance. One person even conjures up a clip on his phone from Salman Khan's hit movie *Jai Ho* (2014) to illustrate his point. Kishore and Vijay are stars in their own right. They epitomise a new bodily ideal for Indian men that is characterised by leanness and muscularity.

## New Middle-Class Professionals

The festival in honour of Ganapati, 'remover of obstacles', brings Mumbai to its knees. Main arteries, flyovers and by-lanes are taken over to transport the idols which, according to local and community-specific customs,[45] need to be submerged in the sea at specific points in time. The seventh and eleventh day of the festival are of special importance, although the city's beaches are busy throughout.

There is an emblematic image of Mumbai: of slowly submerging elephant heads made of plaster, colourfully decorated and garlanded with fragrant flowers. Yet, the actual physical pilgrimage across neighbourhoods and suburbs is something that gets far less attention. It may seem like the city's residents are united in a common pilgrimage to the shore. Yet, in reality, the various groups that make their way across the city have significantly different socioeconomic backgrounds. The same is arguably true for the rest of the year as well, when the city returns to its usual frenetic pace: commuter trains packed to the rafters, sidewalks teeming with business and roads a slow-moving sludge of honking cars.

How do different groups, especially those belonging to the middle class, relate to each other? How do they navigate a changing urban landscape and deal with class difference along the way? And what sort of room for manoeuvrability exists among various middle-class categories? When new middle-class professionals such as Kishore and Vijay make their way across the city, they make another journey too—negotiating the city's social and cultural boundaries. These boundaries shape and add layers to the city; billboards reflect them, buildings resonate with them; and even as everything in rapidly changing India appears to be in flux, some of these borders turn out to be quite robust.

The question that this book enquires into is how young Indians make use of the opportunities that recent economic developments have brought them. It is particularly interested in new middle-class professionals: those who are now employed in professional categories that have emerged out of these developments. Although they may not always feature prominently in more archetypical depictions of the Indian middle class, these men do think of themselves as 'middle class'. However, people I interviewed would frequently employ the term 'new' or 'lower' middle class not only to underline their economic position in relation to other members of the middle class, but also to describe a trajectory of sorts. For one, thinking of themselves as middle class was a decidedly new thing for the parents of these young professionals. Typically, their parents had held working-class jobs themselves before experiencing a trajectory of upward mobility into middle-class ranks at some point. Yet, the relatively new middle class these parents continue to inhabit differs markedly from the one their children aspire to.

Kishore grew up as the son of a labour migrant from Odisha who came to the city to join the textile mills as a weaver. Vijay's father was a low-ranking administrative clerk with the local bureaucracy. They spoke a vernacular language at home (Odia and Hindi respectively), and Marathi with their friends outside. After primary school, their education consisted of private training colleges—notably those offering English-language instruction—or 'simply' on-the-job. While their fathers never made much more than Rs 10,000 per month, they themselves now average ten-fold that. Catering to upper-middle-class clients, they offer personal training sessions across town in upmarket gyms, at clients' homes or in the parks of upscale neighbourhoods.

While their own bodies are crucial to attracting these clients, Kishore and Vijay have also invested in other aspects of their lives. In the roughly ten years that I have known Kishore, I have observed his English improve, his sense of style and fashion change and his general confidence in interacting with those belonging to different socioeconomic strata grow. At the same time, his Chembur upbringing continues to nibble at the carefully delineated peripheries of his new middle-class life. As such, his transition into middle-class ranks is an ongoing project.

## A BOLLYWOOD CONNECTION

Two crucial developments spurred and continue to inform the emergence of the new lean, muscular ideal among Indian men.

The first is the phenomenon whereby Bollywood, Kollywood[46] and other regionally produced movies increasingly come with specific scenes that allow the male hero to flaunt his lean, muscular body. The other is represented by the launch of the Indian edition of *Men's Health* in 2007,[47] and the emergence of other such health and lifestyle magazines that specifically target middle-class men.

It's not easy to say which came first, but both developments draw upon the globalisation of male bodily ideals. Yet, as much as Indian movies or the Indian edition of a foreign-owned magazine appear to build on a globalised momentum, the way these have been appropriated is as locally specific as it is global.[48]

Unlike in Hollywood movies, where actors playing superheroes sport precision-engineered bodies with rock-hard abs,[49] the role male bodies play in Bollywood or other regional Indian cinema is much less likely to build on a functional connection between body-type and the character depicted. This doesn't mean that there is no connection between an actor's body and the movie script. In fact—as interviews with personal trainers of Indian actors revealed—it's often the specific type of muscular body that an actor wishes to portray in a particular movie that sets the agenda and subsequent scripting. The process of transformation the actor undergoes to build such a body is strategically made part of marketing campaigns and can lead to specific training programmes as well as gym and sports brand endorsements. This has a direct impact on the gym floor, where trainers act as brokers of bodily knowledge, translating a particular, fashionable muscular ideal into workout routines, diet plans and related lifestyle choices.

It is important to understand, however, that while such bodies are invariably characterised by their leanness and muscularity, they are not always identically lean or muscular. For instance, actor Farhan Akhtar's depiction of sprinter Milkha Singh in *Bhaag Milkha Bhaag* (2013) was characterised by a leanness and vascularity that was somewhat in keeping with the role he was playing—though decidedly more muscular than Singh himself was during his heyday. For the crime-thriller *Wazir* (2016), in which Akhtar plays an anti-terrorism squad (ATS) officer, he sports a bulkier physique. Even if Akhtar shows relatively little skin in this movie, his strapping frame is clearly visible through his clothes. As various media reports discussed in detail, for *Wazir* he had to adopt a different workout routine and diet plan than for his 2013 hit.[50]

It is striking that reportage on the movie mentions by name his personal trainer—Samir Jaura—whose approaches to bodily transformation have been discussed in various articles in the last few years.[51] There are more and more instances of this kind of direct connection being drawn between actor and celebrity trainer. Bodybuilder and trainer Kris Gethin, for instance, collaborated with Hrithik Roshan for his book on training methods, *The Bodybuilding.com Guide to Your Best Body* (2013). John Abraham provided the foreword for its follow-up, titled *Bollywood Body by Design* (2015).[52]

Especially in Mumbai, newly established, higher-end gyms often boast pictures of Bollywood actors who were present during the opening ceremony or launch of their venue. The walls of a functional training gym in Andheri East (Mumbai) prominently feature pictures of Akshay Kumar, who graced the inauguration and is allegedly passionate about functional training. The gym is operated by Kavita—one of the few female trainers whose career I was able to follow over a long period of time—who is from an English-educated middle-class family from Juhu.

This particular Bollywood connection wouldn't normally be available to a person of her socioeconomic background, but was facilitated by the co-owner of the gym, who works as a marketing manager and used to be one of Kavita's clients. The gym's location in the suburb of Andheri East contributes to the likelihood of movie-industry insiders patronising it. The association between Bollywood stars and gyms, however, isn't location-bound. Across India, gyms collaborate with movie stars, sometimes as brand ambassadors, other times even as investors.

What led Bollywood and regional movie industries to develop such a specific interest and orientation towards the lean, muscular body, spurring the spectacular growth of the Indian fitness industry? While movie heroes have always tended to epitomise a particular masculine ideal, which saw itself partly reflected in powerful 'buff' bodies, this was hardly a specifically sculpted body, at least not in the sense that is common today. Actors such as M.G. Ramachandran (1917–87, Tamil), Dilip Kumar (1922, Hindi) or Mammootty (1951, Malayalam) were undeniably known as ideal-type men, embodying hero-like qualities—yet, their prowess was communicated through body language rather than their actual physiques. The same goes for former Bollywood stars such as Dev Anand (1923–2011), Shammi Kapoor (1931–2011) or Vinod Khanna (1946–2017). Shirtless pictures of these men are rare, if they even exist.

Actor Dharmendra's famous scene in *Pyar Hi Pyar* (1969) is a notable exception. The camera is in thrall to the actor's body, clad in only a towel while he speaks on the phone. Absent from the narrative in this movie and others from this period, however, is a direct connection between the attractive, manly, muscular body and its portrayal as a specific accomplishment of the actor for this particular movie.[53] A noteworthy deviation is the acting career of former wrestler Deedara or Dara Singh (1928–2012). As Seema Sonik Alimchand's biography *Deedara aka Dara Singh* (2016) underscores, this was an actor who did not develop his body as part of his film career, but whose body facilitated this career in the first place. Ronojoy Sen argues in *Nation at Play: A History of Sport in India* (2015)[54] that 'Dara was … the first sportsperson to bring the sporting and the film industry together.'[55]

In an article in *The Indian Quarterly*, filmmaker and columnist Paromita Vohra argues that 'On-screen masculinity could even accommodate decidedly not-good looking men like Pradeep Kumar and Rajendra Kumar, whose appeal is mysterious, or perhaps lies in their being absolutely unthreatening as far as sex appeal goes…' Their bodies are present, but the actors don't have any real bodily presence, so speak. This is something that has clearly changed. The specific scenes within Indian movies that allow for the muscular male body to be showcased in 'all its glory' have become a staple ingredient, and also contribute to an external storyline of transformation. Kollywood blockbuster-actor Vikram, for instance, has made the idea of bodily transformation central to his acting persona. As he explains in Tulsi Badrinath's *Madras, Chennai and the Self: Conversations with the City* (2015):

> 'Every film of mine I have done something. For *Raajapaatai*, I put on size and weight. In *Bhima* I was a fighter, so I worked out and looked like a thug. For *Dhil*, I ate twenty-five egg whites and a whole chicken every day to bulk up.' In *Saamy*, where he played a cop, 'I put on muscle and a paunch.'[56]

Parallels can be drawn here with how 'transformed' bodies fit in with India's rapidly changing urban landscape. On the one hand, these bodies appear intimately connected to the transformation urban India is undergoing; on the other, they seem to exist apart from it. As much as lean, muscular bodies are ubiquitously and indelibly part of popular culture and public spaces—looming from soaring billboards and delivering health and fitness advice in newspapers and magazines—they are also marked by absence. Most men in India, as elsewhere, do not look like this, and most likely never will.

In many ways, Kishore and Vijay 'rule' by absence; their shirtless presence on the final day of Ganesh Chaturthi is a reminder of this. They may elicit desire in other men to look like them, to share their admiration and seek advice. But the promise to become like them is ultimately just that, a promise. Kishore has no illusions about this, though that's not what he communicates to his clients. His business relies on selling a possibility, perhaps even a 'dream'. Thinking of the notion of transformation as merely physical obfuscates the way bodies themselves are layered and imbued with all sorts of meanings. Bollywood provides an insightful window into understanding how bodies are much more than the sum of their bones, muscles, tissue, veins and organs.

## Om Shanti Om

The first movie to explicitly carve out a scene for its lead star to showcase the kind of transformation that would soon become common was Om Shanti Om (2007). In it, Shah Rukh Khan, one of Bollywood's most revered actors, suddenly and rather miraculously sported six-pack abs, a revelation that was widely discussed in the Indian press at the time.

For Kishore, though, the inspiration to build a muscular body came much earlier, from Pyaar Kiya to Darna Kya (1998), which featured the already immensely popular actor Salman Khan. Although the movie and its attendant marketing did not stress a bodily transformation per se—Khan had always been known for being robust and well built—many trainers of Kishore's generation remember it as the first film that sparked their desire for a muscular body.

*Pyaar Kiya … to Darna Kya* is the first mainstream Bollywood production to emphasise its lead actor's body on its movie poster as well as in the song 'O O Jaane Jaana'. During the song, a bare-chested Khan drives down the beach to a makeshift stage, where an elated audience cheers him on. Grabbing a guitar, the actor turns to the crowd to entertain them as the focus remains unavoidably on his powerful chest and abs. Kishore still knows the song by heart, though he probably sports a more defined body than his hero did at the time.

While the muscularity of male bodies has become more pronounced since *Pyaar Kiya to Darna Kya*, there's also a class difference to dissect between this film and *Om Shanti Om*. Salman Khan has always been perceived as a common man's hero, and his physique carries with it decidedly working-class connotations. The appeal of Shah Rukh Khan is decidedly more 'middle class'. This somewhat cursory contrast is reflected in the spatial divide between Chembur (where Kishore grew up and still lives) and Bandra West, which is not just the area Shah Rukh Khan and Salman Khan call home, but also the location of one of the city's best-known Gold's Gyms. At some point, Kishore worked out at this gym to attract well-heeled personal training clients. Engaging in complex routines that involved handstands, pull-ups and various types of push-ups, he envisioned himself performing in front of an audience whose admiration could someday translate to a name within Bollywood. He thought of the expensive membership as an investment, and of himself as working out his way into an imagined future as a high-end trainer to the stars.

The Indian edition of *Men's Health* launched in 2007, the same year *Om Shanti Om* was released. The magazine was widely available at pavement shops across India, right up until its final issue in 2015. Its glossy cover invariably featured a non-famous Indian—usually a fitness enthusiast or personal trainer—whose stunning physique could be achieved by following his training routines as outlined in the magazine. During an interview, the managing editor Jamal Shaikh told me that when the first edition came out, people had a hard time believing that the unknown cover model was actually Indian. The chief editor of the *India Today* group, of which the magazine used to be a part, even demanded to know why he had made use of a foreign model for the launch of the Indian edition.

'He just couldn't believe that these were local models!' Shaikh said. In fact, the first coverline was: 'Indians can have abs too!' Shaikh explained that, at the time, Indian men believed they didn't have the right body-type for developing abs. 'They are vegetarian, they think that will hamper them with building muscles.'[57] Apparently men would show up in such droves for cover shoot call-outs that special security was required to keep them in check. Considering that the magazine never paid its cover models for services rendered, these hopefuls were there for something other than financial gain.

'Abs mean business these days. It's become a sign of achievement,' said Shaikh. 'People equate it with having low body fat. But it is not necessarily healthy. And it is also not always about fitness or endurance.' The magazine conceptualised its covers as communicating different shades of aspiration. 'Sometimes we won't put a six-pack on the cover. Sometimes he will just have four,' Shaikh said. The idea behind this is that 'the guy who will buy the magazine will think "I am better".' But what worked best was success stories. 'Especially those about being overweight and then getting lean, or about those guys who are too thin but want to get bigger.' Admittedly, the magazine featured very few of the latter cases.

It was generally agreed that a lean and muscular look was not enough to make it to the cover. The look had to come with a new fitness routine, something innovative that could be linked to the specific body of the featured model. The cover needed to communicate that between the pages of the issue lay the secret knowledge to achieving such a body. Being aesthetically pleasing wasn't enough, the model also had to be a guide to deeper understanding. These featured bodies were a site of innovation, knowledge and skill. While trainers who were featured thought of the gig as a way to potentially increase their client base, they unknowingly lent their bodies to an evolving discourse on what the lean, muscular body might stand for.

The way Men's Health and its successors present their cover models echoes the way movies craft special scenes for such bodies. The notion of unveiling or even unpacking the body is crucial. The model or actor's body is announced, undressed and subsequently unpacked in the surrounding discussion about what it takes to sculpt and mould oneself into a desirable shape. That readers or moviegoers could potentially achieve the look is the charge underlying each cover or scene with a sense of possibility that feeds into and draws from the narrative of socioeconomic change in India.

## Transformation in a New India

The notion of a 'new' India needs particular examination here.[58] The lean, muscular body is not only held possible within the context of a new India, but also epitomises it. I engage with the colonial legacy in detail later on—especially in terms of British imperial perspectives on the emasculated or effeminate Hindu body (see chapter three). But what I want to dwell on first is the very notion of a trajectory.

There is a new bodily ideal, true, but the very focus on the male body is novel as well. Whereas previously men were the ones observing women, judging their bodies and setting standards for attractiveness, their own 'male' bodies have now become the object of the gaze as well. However, the male body is principally one that is scrutinised by other men. While *Men's Health* and similar lifestyle magazines use bare-chested models to portray a more 'attractive' body, and Bollywood heroes make heroines swoon with their dance routines, ultimately they are all selling a highly specific bodily ideal—and they are selling it to other men.

Globally, *Men's Health* and comparable magazines primarily cater to a male readership. Muscular actors who portray superheroes in Hollywood blockbusters also frequently discuss their workout and dietary regimes in popular media, setting the tone for new such routines *for* men. What makes the Indian case so specific, however, is the wider socioeconomic context in which these developments take shape. Leaving aside popular narratives of economic growth and concomitant social change, there is no denying that the Indian context is also coloured by underdevelopment, rampant inequality, poverty and malnourishment. There is plenty of evidence for the limitations and exclusivity of India's newness discourse.

The construction of a new India is essentially an incomplete process, something that is still ongoing, and that conceivably will never reach an 'end stage'. This is personified by the country's ever-looming building sites, road constructions and multiplying critical issues (many the product of its bulging population numbers). On the other hand, perhaps this incompleteness comes with the way the idea of this modern nation builds (metaphorically as well as literally) on the notion of transformation. The body is a particularly rich site to tease out the broader implications of this transformation, with regard to the position its middle classes take up within this trajectory and the way India relates to the outside world. How can we understand this hazy macro-reality in relation to the micro-realities of the everyday? How do the bodies of trainers, bodybuilders and clients relate to the socioeconomics of a rapidly changing urban landscape? When it comes to economic, social or cultural change, the body enacts these changes and is changed by them too. Obesity, diabetes and related issues, for example, are the outcome of changing diets, the availability of readymade products, the overconsumption of carbohydrates and sugar, and the product of once active but now predominantly sedentary lifestyles. At the same time, the body is never just a receptor but always also an actor: one that makes decisions and actively engages with its changing environment. It is guided by ideas and notions of health, aesthetics and, perhaps most of all, influenced by the gaze of others. The body is in dialogue with its environment and reflects what goes on in society.

The implied dichotomy between an old and a new India, or a developing versus underdeveloped one, is therefore less interesting than the way newness itself is experienced. Everyday 'middle-class' lives also function irrespective of the framing narratives of old India–new India. As fast as developments in India appear to be—the proliferation of shopping malls, the spectacular growth of the fitness industry, and the availability of goods and services previously unheard of—change can also seem sluggish as bureaucratic hurdles remain seemingly the same, regular power cuts are inevitable and issues with water pressure insistent.

As with bodies in the gym, on a bench press pushing weights, in front of the mirror with dumb-bells, or positioned for another round on the leg press, actual progress is often more measured than the narrative of change would imply. Bodies transform slowly, indolently, often without much result at all. This is what Kishore also remarked after a group training session that he had invited me to observe. 'It took me a lot of time to build this body,' he said as he rubbed his abs through his T-shirt. Dedication and discipline had been key, but genetics and a certain body type had benefited him as well.

To a certain degree, his bodily transformation, specifically his body language, also mirrors the socioeconomic change he has effectuated as an increasingly higher-end trainer. Genetics notwithstanding, his own working-class background was not particularly conducive to this. Unlike his career trajectory, or the smoothness of his bodily transformation, Kishore's journey of upward social and cultural mobility has been a bumpy one.

The many reflections on the idea of the middle class in popular media and in academic publications rarely consider what it means to those who belong to this group. While the adjectives of lower, middle and upper slot people in more narrowly defined categories, there are no conclusive descriptors for defining the 'old' or 'new' middle classes. Those who self-identify as upper middle class generally use the adjective 'new' to refer to those they perceive as 'lower'. Lower does not necessarily correspond to 'less money' but instead a briefer history of belonging to the middle classes.

Family histories tend to reveal a generational understanding of what this middle-class belonging entails. Young professionals I spoke to in the information technology (IT) industry, working for Wipro or Infosys, would frequently narrate their families' trajectories in terms of their own education—for instance, attending convent school, and thus receiving almost all their education in English—but also the educational and professional histories of their parents, and even grandparents.[59] Although they spoke a language other than English at home, these software engineers and their parents were very comfortable with English. They described their parents as 'educated'; their mothers were teachers or government servants, their fathers took care of a family business or were accountants, doctors, engineers or lawyers. Most grandmothers were homemakers, but sometimes a grandmother would also be described as an 'educated woman', 'traditional ... but intelligent nonetheless'. A certain conflation of class and caste and notions of religiosity percolated such recollections. Upper-middle-classness could be understood as a privileged, though not necessarily elite,[60] position in society.

What actually separates lower from middle and middle from upper? As much as it makes sense to seek all-encompassing definitions, especially considering the numbers involved, it makes more sense to focus on the mobile trajectories of those who navigate and negotiate these categories. It is important to treat these categories as inherently flexible and negotiable, despite what those who belong to each might say. People often defend their own middle-class position, presumably against those who seek upward mobility and might one day consider themselves part of the establishment.

The context of India's changing urban landscape provides opportunities to new middle-class professionals like Kishore and Vijay: the transformation of urban space has the potential to destabilise old and entrenched hierarchies. It makes everything a lot less certain.

## A Chembur Gym Rat

At heart Kishore remains a typical Chembur boy, as he would describe himself, having lived in the same locality of Mumbai all his life. His father arrived from Odisha to join the cotton mills of Parel in the 1970s, working there until the 1980s, when the mills ceased operations. He held various odd jobs and, as long as Kishore can remember, life was characterised by financial precarity. His father's last earned salary of Rs 7,000 contrasts significantly with the Rs 1 lakh[61] Kishore himself makes as a personal trainer. He describes the home he grew up in as 'nothing more than a hut', though the family now lives in a ground-floor apartment on a tree-lined street, which his earnings have paid for.

Kishore completed all of his schooling as well as his B.Com. in Chembur but admits that studying was never his forte. Instead, he was the 'sporty guy' in school, the one who excelled at all games. An old classmate of his said he was always 'running around the neighbourhood', and that she couldn't remember a time when he was 'not working on his muscles'. She and other childhood friends are impressed by how he never let his 'humble origins' stand in the way of making something of his life, not just his muscles.

When I met Kishore for the first time, now almost a decade ago, he picked me up on his bike in front of Bandra's Gold's Gym and we drove off to Band Stand on the sea-facing promenade. A throng of mainly adolescent men would gather there, eagerly awaiting the rare appearance of Salman Khan on his apartment's balcony, a 'tradition' which would repeat itself every Sunday. Their anticipation was not so much for the actor's appearance, but about whether or not he would take his shirt off and flex his muscles. Shah Rukh Khan was not known to entertain such fancies in a similar way and usually kept himself secluded in his mansion, just a few hundred metres down the road.

Sitting on the rocks facing the sea, Kishore and I listened to the voices of the crowd bubbling with excitement. He knew from experience that the actor rarely showed himself, and rumour had it he was actually abroad on a movie shoot. Yet the place was important to him, not least because of the influence his hero had had on his own trajectory. Growing up in a working-class environment, schooling was deemed important but earning money and becoming self-reliant even more so. When Kishore was sixteen, an uncle invited him to join his packaging business, a job which helped his family make ends meet but held little promise for the future.

Influenced by Salman Khan's *Pyaar Kiya* ... Kishore had started working out at a local gym, where he rapidly made a name for himself because of the gains he was making. He soon had a loyal following of enthusiastic local 'gym rats' who consulted him on their own gym routines, which led the gym owner to offer Kishore a job. Though it was a poorly equipped gym that catered to a local working-class crowd, it allowed him to make his first forays into the world of fitness. He quickly understood he needed to invest more if he wanted to move up the ladder and turn his passion into a stable source of income.

Kishore realised that working out was becoming more popular among those with 'more money to spend' and could lead to employment in gyms in well-heeled neighbourhoods. As he started exploring better career options, the industry itself was becoming more professional as well. Gyms were no longer the working-class places they had once been; they were becoming better equipped and had begun offering a whole array of health-related services. Like Café Coffee Days ('CCDs'), fashion outlets of American brands such as Levi's and Nike, and fast-food restaurants, gyms were 'suddenly' everywhere, Kishore remembers.

## CITY PERMEATES BODY

India's urban landscape has undergone an incontrovertible transformation since the new millennium, with burgeoning spaces of consumption and leisure that specifically target the ever-expanding middle classes. The city permeates the body not just physically through its orifices[62]—the large quantities of air pollution, the skin soaking up dust, arteries clogged with abundantly available cheap snacks, the ever-present danger of dengue and other types of viral diseases—but also mentally and as such socially and culturally. Considering the inherently diffuse nature of Indian urban space, with its constant surge of newcomers, the body has come to be a marker of difference, and almost literally a vessel of social and cultural mobility. As the ever-present body traverses the city, moving in and out of different situations and locations, it carries with it meanings well beyond its immediate physical appeal.

Kishore's involvement in English language courses in small institutes of variable quality across the city, doing various accreditation courses with fitness training institutes, and the gyms he has been involved with at over time, all add up to a trajectory in which he has not only worked on his body but also the 'packaging', so to speak.

His English has improved remarkably since our first conversation at Band Stand. These days, his relative fluency is put to good use on his regular Facebook and Instagram updates, through which he advertises his services and connects with potential clients. In such updates, he portrays a bodily confidence that appeals to potential upper-middle-class clients who seek his guidance in developing their own bodies. In these posts, I have known him to play with a dash of working-class bravura, which also holds a certain appeal (albeit in moderation) to potential clients. This is more difficult to comprehend than the ostensive appeal of his body. His natural exuberance is laced with a harder edge, which some might describe as rowdy or even aggressive. The hint of his working-class upbringing adds to Kishore's persona as a self-made man, exuding a masculinity defined by survival and overcoming the odds.

It is clear, however, that Kishore's Chembur appeal is limited to the actual workout sessions. He is aware that his clients will never quite consider him their equal or make him fully part of their private lives. Even though he is doing well as a personal trainer, his salary wouldn't necessarily permit him to hire *himself* for the services he renders either. In that sense, his clients belong to a different socioeconomic stratum altogether. But there is more yet to this difference. Kishore's trajectory from working class into lower-middle-class terrain, from being educated in a vernacular language to having entered the workforce at a young age, is not a pathway his clients would ever consider for themselves or their children. Their education will invariably have been in English, probably at a convent school with a network of similarly positioned people. The kind of sociocultural capital this provides from early on feeds into the less tangible difference between positions within the middle class. Kishore's upward trajectory is marked by seeking to close an economic gap as well as a social and cultural one.

## MAYBE WE ARE GOONDAS!

After inspecting a number of pandals across Chembur, and stopping to pick up some cheap whisky at a small shack, we gradually make our way back to Khardev Nagar in Chembur. We park the motorcycles at a safe distance from the party, which has grown considerably in size since we left. A neatly dressed gentleman approaches and identifies himself as a police officer in civilian clothes. Although I am unable to follow the discussion, it is abundantly clear that he wants both Kishore and Vijay to put their shirts back on. They begrudgingly agree. However, the moment the officer is out of sight, they immediately take off their shirts again.

Vijay explains that 'the guy thinks we're trouble-makers', to which Kishore adds 'goondas',[63] shrugging his powerful shoulders. 'He thinks we're crooks, man,' Vijay says and laughs. 'Maybe we are,' he adds. 'We're kings of this world man!' He high-fives Kishore. Vijay pats his chest and turns to me. 'That guy is nothing, man, forget him.' Taking a swig of his whisky-and-Coke, he says: 'He's a nobody, that's what he is. A nobody!' He wants to know my opinion but it has all happened so fast that I can't quite make up my mind. Why not simply wear your shirts if it might get you into trouble this way? 'This is our day to shine,' Kishore says. 'We live all year for this.' He points at the party going on further down the street. 'It's our moment of glory.'

Walking back, I wonder what they mean. Aren't both shining all the time, assisting clients in their workout routines, participating in bodybuilding competitions such as MuscleMania, and posting pictures of themselves in various poses online? What precisely makes this moment stand out? Perhaps because they are able to 'show off' in their own neighbourhood for a change?

Vijay's personal history sheds light on something crucial: upward trajectories always carry the indelible impression of one's background into one's future. He grew up in the same locality as Kishore and, like him, has integrated his Chembur 'heritage' into how he 'markets' himself and his physical accomplishments. But this narrative is not easy to control, nor is it a simple thing to pick and choose what aspects from the past to retain and what he should keep at a remove.

Vijay's father, who is deceased, held a job with the municipal corporation for most of his life. With a brother employed with a logistics company and an elder sister who is a software engineer, the family has a longer history of thinking of itself as middle class than Kishore's does. Vijay's father's clerical position helped in this. Even though Vijay's English is more fluent than Kishore's, it would be a mistake to think that he benefited from superior education. He too has mainly 'improved' on his English along the way. At nineteen, he completed a diploma in hotel management and was hired as a bartender by the Ritz-Carlton in the UK where he worked for a year and a half. He returned to Mumbai for a brief spell and was subsequently hired to work for a five-star hotel in Dubai, which eventually facilitated a transfer to the US.

But Vijay's heart was never in the hospitality business. 'To join a hotel was just an excuse. I didn't want to work there.' His main goal was to travel, to see the world. While working out in the hotel gym, he met 'some army recruiters' and was convinced to enlist. 'They told me about this new plan; if you are a foreign national and can speak good English and can speak a foreign language, then you can join the army and get citizenship.' A degree of some sort was also required, and to be good in sports—something that had gotten him noticed in the first place. Vijay explained that he joined 'the rangers battalion, infantry', but was always a little vague about what precisely was expected of him in the army, perhaps because of enlistment regulations which limited how much he could say about it.

Once, talking about his time in the US Army, he said: 'Was real, real shit, man. Wasn't intelligent stuff; jump from plane, get out of the helicopter, use rope, mountain trekking.' But the pay was good, he insisted. His first trip took him to Afghanistan for nine months, but none of what he was made to do there was particularly brave, he feels—'that's just in the movies'. He was also stationed in Europe for a joint exercise of three months, during which he visited Germany, Poland, Lithuania and Latvia. It gave him the kind of international exposure that somebody from Chembur could only have dreamt about, he felt.

Now a US Army Reserve, which requires him to return to the country on a regular basis, Vijay spends most of his time with Kishore, attending to personal training clients and taking care of his family. As a personal trainer, he charges around

Rs 20,000 per month, which includes four one-on-one sessions per week. The price is high-end, and if he is completely booked, his income could average as much as Rs 2 lakh per month. This rarely happens, since clients come and go and sessions often get cancelled. He describes his clients as 'very rich, high-class people ... richest class of people'. He wouldn't even refer to them as middle class, as he puts it.

Besides knowledge of training techniques, such clients 'need well-spoken people to come to their house to train', Vijay says. His army qualifications certainly help here, but also his fluency in English and the fact that he's well-travelled. During the Ganesh Chaturthi celebrations, he flexed his muscles to underline that ultimately that's what his clients see, of course. 'But they like it that I have been in the army, they think I am the commando-shit or something.' He makes considerably more than most of his peers in Chembur, and believes that the next step is to become a celebrity trainer, catering to Bollywood clients. 'Otherwise I can always go back to the States, join the army again.'

## SHINING ALL THE TIME IN INDIA

The moment of interruption by the police officer points to the complexity of Kishore and Vijay's trajectories. Sometime after the Ganesh Chaturthi celebrations, I asked Vijay what precisely the police officer had been after, and it emerged that there was more to the story than I had been told then. A few years earlier, Kishore and Vijay had been involved in collecting loans for a local politician and businessman. As a result, both had made their share of enemies in Chembur. It had even led to a kerfuffle between members of two opposing gangs, something that had resulted in the two spending time in jail the previous year.

'We knocked out all of them, two broken arms, two in ICU,' Vijay told me over the phone one evening. Allegedly, the case for self-defence had not worked out, and they had been found guilty of various charges related to aggression and violence. It wasn't the first fight the two had been involved in. During a 'bigger one', Vijay had been stabbed in his side. The scar, he felt, added to his carefully cultivated fighter persona and helped secure 'elite' clients for his personalised outdoor training routines. He had also stabbed some people himself, he emphasised. 'Big fight, man!' This fight had also led to some jail time. Vijay claims the cops involved were corrupt, but adds, 'I am not saying it wasn't my mistake at all.' He was 'too young' those days. Coming back to the incident during Ganesh Chaturthi he noted: 'These cops want to fight me all over.' Because of their muscular bodies, he feels, they are automatically suspicious.

While these stories involve serious violence and aggression, casting the duo as goonda muscle men, they also need to be understood in a larger context. Neighbourhoods such as Chembur, which are still known as working class, even if gentrification has permeated there (see chapter four), are part of a city in motion. Its inhabitants can't always boast pristine, unsullied trajectories from A to B to C. Like some of the men described later in this book, who have resorted to the use of anabolic steroids and growth hormones, the health and fitness narratives they share about themselves and 'sell' to their clients are not necessarily tainted by the details of their journeys. Part of the appeal of contracting Kishore or Vijay for their services may very well be their working-class Chembur backgrounds, laced with references to violence and aggression.

As we join the party, several men are in the process of getting a pick-up truck ready to transport the idol to Dadar. It is around seven o'clock; the sun has set and the temperature is gradually becoming more bearable, though the intense dancing has left many exhausted and drenched in sweat. The steel contraption against which the idol rests has some space on top, and Kishore indicates that I should climb there and position myself behind Ganesha's left ear so that I can sit and watch the crowds from above as we commence on our snail-paced journey across town. He himself will be on the cart too, not just to keep the God company but also to claim his own stage.

As much as Ganesha is known to be the remover of obstacles, we will have to negotiate quite a few on the way, not least because the height of our transport is such that we will have to take the idol off the cart and carry it underneath a number of flyovers. For most of the route, Vijay either walks alongside or sits on the outer edge, chatting with Kishore's family members or friends, or glancing at the screen of his mobile phone. He has a personal training session scheduled for seven o'clock in the morning the next day, but his client has requested an earlier time because of a meeting and the maddening traffic from Andheri West (where his client resides) to his office in Worli. It is one of the reasons Vijay does not want to drink too much tonight. However, I also know that he is less than keen to accompany us all the way to Dadar, which in his experience might take longer than is optimistically expected.

As we slope through traffic, it is slowly sinking in that our initial speedy progress has gradually been reduced to a casual walking speed. The Khardev Nagar party is now part of a never-ending parade of similar carts, all bedecked with colossal Ganesha statues in various shapes and poses, seemingly pushed forward by the relentless exclamations of *Ganapati Bappa Morya*,[64] occasionally followed by a *Pudchya Varshi Laukar Ya*. Seen from on top, the suburbs all blend into one as thousands of people throng the streets to watch the carts snake by. Our path cuts across socioeconomic differences, while the flyovers are physical reminders of the city's ongoing negotiation with economic developments, population growth and the limitations of its narrow land mass.

When we come to a near standstill, I climb down the contraption I have spent the better part of three hours on top of, and make my way to a public restroom I spotted from above. Vijay follows suit, the whisky now as good as finished, but the road ahead still long. Afterwards, while buying a bottle of water at one of the roadside stalls, I notice the truck suddenly moving and speeding up. Vijay has already started running to catch up, but the incline of the flyover is too steep and the truck too fast, and we quickly lose sight of our party altogether. On a nearly deserted flyover, we continue jogging along, me barely keeping up with Vijay, who hardly seems to notice that he is jogging at all, and who is also hurriedly talking to Kishore on his phone. Half an hour later, we manage to catch up with our party when it gets stuck in another jam near Shivaji Park, theoretically within spitting distance of Dadar Beach.

I clamber on top of the truck and try to count the number of carts ahead of us, all heading for the same seashore to immerse their idols in Mahim Bay. Vijay says his goodbyes, realising that this may be his last chance of catching an auto home. He has taken part in this procession numerous times and knows that, although we are close, it will be a number of hours before we actually reach. Removing his shirt from his belt and putting it back on, he asks if I am sure I want to stay. Since I have come all this way, I feel I may as well see it through till the end. He smiles, gets into an auto and heads off, checking his phone for messages from tomorrow's clients.

## SUBMERGING GANESHA, IMMERGING IN THE CITY

Multiple bands are now joining up, keeping up a rhythm that contrasts with the flagging energy of the people on the carts. It has been a long road, yet there is no choice but to continue dancing and singing along a little longer. Kishore is still in his usual spot, encouraging his fellow community members to keep the spirit alive, not unlike the way he conducts his training sessions. However, the road ahead is a clogged artery that no amount of diet advice can unblock.

I climb on top of the truck and am joined by two of Kishore's neighbourhood friends, who have been part of the festivities throughout and seem to be in need of a break. They have known Kishore since childhood, and although they admire his stamina and perseverance, they also find his efforts to continuously motivate others to keep the spirit alive somewhat amusing. We stand up to admire and photograph a beautifully decorated truck with an incredibly large following of worshippers—all dressed in white, though festively blemished by coloured powder.

Kishore's friends are keen to share their stories with me: one studies accounting, the other has just joined his father's real estate business after a brief spell in IT. Their paths relate to growing up within the limitations of Chembur but also speak of upward socioeconomic mobility; personal histories that, however brief, are themselves coloured or patterned by the changing socioeconomic conditions of India.

They are middle class, but with the qualifiers of 'new' or 'lower'. Neither would make the mistake of thinking of himself as upper middle class. Their awareness of their relative position in society is as crystal clear as the water we are approaching is muddy, having witnessed countless immersions over the past few days.

As we approach the beach, instructions and regulations, enforced by a heavy police presence, become more pronounced to facilitate a speedy transition from cart to water. Kishore, with some others, lifts the immense statue off the cart and carries it to the sea. The auspicious moment is marked by a wave of fatigue and relief washing over the crowd.

Ultimately, Kishore and company were not able to carry the idol very far into the water. The size and balance of the statue was such that it quickly tumbled over, giving in to its inevitable descent. By the time Kishore emerged from the water, the next party's Ganesha was halfway under. With nothing left to do and exhaustion rampant, the party quickly gathered on top of the cart—decidedly more spacious with the departure of the main guest—and headed back to Chembur. I was staying in Bandra West then, so I walked down Old Cadell Road, or Swatantrya Veer Savarkar Road, as it is now known, against better judgement hoping to find a taxi.

Late at night, India's beating heart—which never sleeps, and certainly not on the final day of Ganesh Chaturthi—was surprisingly quiet. In the distance, the crescendo of drum bands could be heard, its strength lessening and the lights still on in buildings nearby diminishing. As I finally found a taxi driver to take me along, I realised that the city would soon return to its normal chaotic self. In this city, Kishore and Vijay would recommence their roles as trainers, offering their clients a way to deal with 'all' that new India had in store for them. The adulation received from the audience would have to wait for another year, though. As much as their bodies are crucial to their upward trajectories, the public unveiling by taking off their shirts earlier could also be thought of as a symbolic reminder of the constraints society will continue to put in these men's way.

# CHAPTER 2

# A SMALL NEIGHBOURHOOD GYM

*Once through this ruined city did I pass*
*I espied a lonely bird on a bough and asked*
*'What knowest thou of this wilderness?'*
*It replied: 'I can sum it up in two words:*
*'Alas, Alas!'*

– Khushwant Singh, *Delhi*

A grey haze greets me as I step out of the house. The hesitant morning sun does its best to percolate through, and the result is a pinkish sky that is something between vaguely charming and disturbingly apocalyptic. The air is redolent of something metallic, the smell of which competes with garbage scattered around and the burning of heaps of leaves. The neighbourhood is basking in an idyllic quietude interrupted only by the distant honking of cars and autos. The houses in CR Park in South Delhi are generally tall—three to four storeys high—with significant fences topped by pointy spikes, as well as the occasional guard indolently parked on a plastic chair. Cars line the streets: Maruti Suzuki DZires, Tata Indigos and the occasional four-wheel drive or Jaguar, washed dutifully by the guards or by boys who patrol the neighbourhood offering their services. The battle against dust, however, seems lost from the onset.

Two men of indeterminable age are out for a brisk walk, one sporting a turban and fierce moustache, the other balding, a ring of dyed black hair all that is left of what must have been a head-full once. He occasionally uses an old blue towel draped around his neck to wipe the sweat off his face, adroitly removing his heavy-set black-rimmed glasses without missing a beat in the story he is enthusiastically sharing. I take a left into a nearby lane and squeeze through the narrow opening in the gate. It is left ajar during the day but kept resolutely shut at night, this narrow side-gate the only way in or out. Security is taken very seriously in CR Park, as is the case in all of South Delhi.

The city has a history of unrest turning gruesomely violent, and even though this does not necessarily set it apart from other Indian cities, the inner suburbs of Delhi continue to be characterised by imposing yellow gates. Especially at night, when the gates are shut, it can be quite a challenge to find one's way to a particular address. These residential areas continue to be referred to rather euphemistically as 'colonies', something which has its origin in the post-Independence resettlements. As Rana Dasgupta writes in *Capital: The Eruption of Delhi* (2014), Delhi's bizarre vocabulary of residential residences, with its associated social and security paranoia, 'says much about what people in this city expect from home: they live in *housing societies* and *estates* which are contained in *blocks*, themselves sub-divisions of *sectors, enclaves* and *colonies*'.[65] These colonies have long gelled into one distinctly upmarket enclave that people now often simply refer to as South Delhi.

Internal differences in terms of the sociocultural backgrounds of the inhabitants of these colonies have gradually diminished as well. While CR Park is still known as a predominantly Bengali area—its well-known fish market continues to thrive because of this—there is no denying that it has stopped being solely Bengali. Its upper-middle-class identity remains resolutely intact, however, as is the case with its adjacent neighbourhoods such as Greater Kailash (GK), parts I and II. The relative quietude, the men out for a brisk stroll, white socks determinedly pulled up to their knees, the brand-new cars awaiting their regular bath, all reek of this upper-middle-classness.

However, if one were to ask the inhabitants of CR Park to define what precisely this designation of upper middle class means, the answers would likely vary considerably. The possession of landed property figures into such accounts, financial wealth, of course, but equally I found people stressing their ability to speak English, their level of education and, related to this, their history and experience with education itself; parents and even grandparents having attended higher education, children enrolled in English-medium private education, and the occasional family member with a schoolbook or biography to their name. Those in CR Park would never think of themselves as *new* middle class; those are decidedly 'other' people. However, tales of middle class belonging tend to be of a slippery, fluidic quality, and CR Park is no exception. What exactly middle-class belonging entails is often a matter of individual interpretation.

## SLOWING INDIA DOWN

The Mumbai suburb of Chembur, where I met Kishore and Vijay for the Ganapati celebrations in the previous chapter, continues to be known as a working-class neighbourhood. Yet, the trajectories of the two trainers have been decidedly upwardly mobile in socioeconomic terms—something that is reflected in their physical mobility across Mumbai, providing personal training to clients in elite neighbourhoods such as Andheri East, Bandra West or Malabar Hill.

This chapter focuses on the trainers and clients of a small neighbourhood gym called BodyHolics in South Delhi. But first, let's continue a little longer on the walk this chapter opened with. For a period of nine months between 2013 and 2014, I made this walk almost every day. This was a relatively short walk, about fifteen minutes, compared to the much longer ones I would embark on in various Indian cities over the years to map and 'experience' urban change. These walks, both short and long, raised serious reservations about the idea that India was indeed changing 'incredibly fast'. Walking from South Delhi to Gurgaon, or exploring the outer limits of Noida on foot, I often found myself reflecting on the speed of this change.

Such walks would take me from Chennai's outer-lying new middle-class suburb of Pallikaranai to the far more bohemian, upper-middle-class Besant Nagar; from the shady lanes of Koramangala, a popular suburb for well-heeled software engineers in Bangalore, to the iconic MG Road in the heart of the city; and from Mumbai's breezy sea-facing suburbs to its swelteringly hot interior ones. Walking, the slowest mode of transportation, challenged the speed at which I had assumed India was changing. In fact, often on such walks, reflecting on the personal histories that informants had shared with me, I could not help conclude that change was also incredibly slow.

## Negotiating Traffic, Crossing Boundaries

I squeeze through the narrow gate on my usual morning walk to the gym, reaching a road almost permanently clogged with impatient traffic. It is a few weeks before Diwali and it has become noticeably colder in the past few days. Some of the stray dogs, who usually congregate near the stall of a chaiwallah, are now wearing jackets against the chill as they rummage through a pile of refuse carved out of the plastic bags dumped on this street corner. The tea seller himself is smoking a beedi and checking his battered old Nokia for messages. Casually, an auto driver leans against the back of his rickshaw, sipping a cup of steaming chai. A vegetable seller navigates his cart around it, loudly calling attention to his merchandise, but drawing only the interest of the pack of strays. Momentarily stepping into the midst of the slow-moving traffic in order to avoid the holes that pockmark the sidewalk, as well as the various stalls selling snacks, paan and calling cards that take up what is left of the space between, I make my way to the extraordinarily busy Outer Ring Road that runs in front of BodyHolics.

The T-junction that merges with this road is flanked by colourful billboards advertising private education at various institutions across the city, and even more visually striking advertisements suggesting solutions for hair loss, obesity and other health-related issues. One faded billboard shows the before and after of a man who has lost considerable weight due to an Ayurveda-inspired intervention, while a more recent one offers hope to women, who look like they have gotten an early start on the season's sweets, that they too could be shaadi-ready.[66] This is a regular topic of discussion among the female clients of BodyHolics. The ready availability of fast food, the demands of social life with its never-ending string of parties and weddings, and, most of all, sedentary lifestyles all contribute to the risk of putting on weight. This is a concern that is shared by the gym's male clients as well, though they are more likely to discuss it in terms of wanting to look fit. While the latest muscular looks of Bollywood heroes may be a source of inspiration for the younger members that turn up in the evening, a majority of the men who attend the gym in the morning are in their late twenties or older, and in general married. They are concerned first and foremost with budding potbellies that remind them of their fathers and of the health advice they have received about the risk of diabetes.

As I bide my chance to cross the ring road, I notice some regular clients entering BodyHolics. The gym offers valet car parking, though this does not amount to much more than that there is a person who manages the double-parking issue that cannot be avoided on the relatively small strip in front of the entrance. I spot one of the morning's regulars leaning against his car, the door open, some paperwork spread open on the passenger seat, busily discussing something on his phone. Phones regularly interrupt morning workouts at the gym. In general, clients carry one or two with them, either keeping them with them during their workout, or leaving them charging on the small desk near the entrance where they will regularly congregate to check for messages. Most are business owners or managers, and there never seems to be a break from their urgently required involvement in pressing matters.

## A Gym's Rhythm and Sounds

The moment I open the BodyHolics door, I'm hit by a blast of Bollywood music that overpowers the honking of cars outside. On the gym floor itself, this music competes with the sound of weights being casually tossed on top of each other as well as the loud grunting emanating from Sunil's throat as he bench-presses a weight equal to that of Ravi, the head trainer who is assisting him. It is a spartanly decorated gym that could have used a major overhaul some time ago. However, due to a conflict between the building's owner and the gym's two managers, general maintenance and repairs have fallen behind. The first time I visited it, I was rather surprised to see how busy it was, considering that competition abounds in South Delhi. In walking vicinity of my home in CR Park there were at least six other gyms, while nearby Saket (Select Citywalk mall) and East of Kailash (right next to the subway station) were home to branches of globally operating chains Fitness First and Gold's Gym. Most BodyHolics members had been regulars for a few years already, and as a result, seemed to know each other well, living in the neighbourhood and spending free time together outside the gym. The rather desperate state of some of the equipment did not seem to bother them as long as the personalised service continued.

Gyms come with their own rhythm, and BodyHolics was no exception to this. While its morning shift was characterised by the coming and going of local businessmen, their wives and the occasional manager working for some multinational, evenings drew a younger, student-aged crowd. The gym was open from six o'clock in the morning until noon, closing for a few hours to give its trainers some respite. More or less the same battalion of trainers returned in the late afternoon to assist the evening crowd until ten o'clock. Since the gym offered personalised training to all its members, there was considerable interaction between clients and staff, not just about workout routines but also all sorts of related and unrelated topics.

I notice Amit and Supriya, one of his clients, watching one of the TV screens mounted on the wall above. The somewhat disapproving look on Supriya's face contrasts markedly with that of Amit, who seems enthralled. The TV is, as usual, tuned to MTV India, and the hit song 'Tattad Tattad' from the movie *Goliyon Ki Raasleela Ram-Leela*, a runaway success in the cinemas. The movie opens with actor Ranveer Singh arriving on a motorcycle, lying down on it, dressed in embroidered jeans, a tight-fitting purple shirt, cell phone in hand, nonchalantly cruising through a Gujarati make-believe, fairy-tale bazaar, where he is joined by rowdy-looking men, all dressed in yellow kurtas and matching turbans. It is hardly the most original way to introduce a lead character in a Bollywood movie—virtually all male leads have a few iconic arrival-on-motorcycle scenes to their name[67]—but the casualness with which Ranveer reclines on his motorcycle, at some point even flipping his cell phone from one hand to the other in order to take a selfie, is over-the-top even by industry standards.

Once the motorcycle comes to a halt, the men zoom up to the lead actor, then scatter to their designated positions to start the opening dance routine. Ranveer[68] emerges from the crowd, his purple shirt fully unbuttoned, sporting well-defined six-pack abs. Soon the actor is being carried through the crowd on what looks like a wooden board, possibly a door. Frenetically dancing, thrusting his crotch upward to a pulsating rhythm, Ranveer's moves are an inebriant to the crowd. When his posse of dancers pass a balcony on which four traditionally dressed women are slowly losing their minds, the actor takes off his shirt, flaunts his muscular physique, and even strikes a few bodybuilding poses. Overcome by the visual spectacle, one of the women on the balcony faints, while Ranveer continues to dance, this time surrounded by a group of women keen to take his picture and cosy up to him. The video is deeply erotic, yet full of religious signifiers: images of Shiva decorate the walls, and various extras are dressed as Krishna, Ram and Hanuman, suggestive of a divine sanctioning of all that is so scrumptiously on display. While this is hardly bhakti poetry,[69] the scene is suffused with adulation and devotion.

As a floor trainer, Amit does not come close to meeting the lean, muscular ideal that Ranveer Singh exemplifies. A solidly built, muscular 'Jat-boy',[70] he has been employed with BodyHolics for a little over a year. He enjoys working out himself, but the muscularity Ranveer Singh displays in his movie would require Amit to make an investment in his body that he currently does not have the money nor time for. This particular morning, he is not only responsible for Supriya's workout, but simultaneously for a number of other clients who all rely on him to tell them what exercises to do next, as well as to listen to their physical complaints, provide dietary advice and also basically be a listening ear to anything they want to share. The Bollywood videos that provide these workouts with a soundtrack are a reminder of the gym culture's source of inspiration, as much as they underline 'failure', since hardly any of the members—or, indeed, the trainers—sport a Ranveer-like body.

## MEETING BODILY IDEALS

In 2013, the *Hindustan Times* ran a 'Get Healthy, Delhi' campaign, which featured 'ordinary' Delhiites who had taken a pledge to get fit. One Saturday, the paper ran a large article titled 'Kisme Kitna Hai Dum' (Who Is the Strongest), about two businessmen who 'say their biggest weakness is food' and were pitted against each other in a face-off to see who could lose more fat.[71] Accompanied by a set of vivid pictures, the battle was a cheerful one, but its ultimate goal was to warn against a serious and fast-growing problem in India: obesity and associated problems such as diabetes and hypertension.

The two businessmen are in many ways interchangeable with the male clients who frequent BodyHolics. It's up to the floor trainers to come up with a workout for the day, often specifically tuned to one or two areas of the body. For these clients, life is hectic and time short; most run construction businesses and spend the bulk of their day stuck in snail-paced traffic from one building site to another. It is this dilemma that magazines such as *Men's Health* tap into when they discuss the benefits of a lean and muscular body. Ultimately, however, this body is an ideal type. For the majority of middle-class men, the challenge will be exactly the one so jovially illustrated by the *Hindustan Times*: reducing fat levels and potentially avoiding associated ailments.

Twenty-three-year-old Ratish, one of the gym's regulars, was one of the few whose strapping figure came close to the Ranveer ideal. When he stood in front of the mirror flexing his muscles, the floor trainers whose focus should be on the gym's clients, immediately shifted to what was on display: heavily pronounced pectoral muscles, sharply defined triceps, bulging biceps and a V-shaped back. Recently having finished a degree in hotel management from an elite institute in Switzerland, Ratish moved back to Delhi in search of a job and clearly came from a well-off family. In the morning, we would usually briefly catch up and the floor trainers, whose English was limited, often tried to participate in our conversations. Ratish interlaced his stories with rapid Hindi, but he lacked the slang that lubricated the bolder tales of the trainers.

When Ratish walked in, the general manager, Manish, usually quickly emerged from his office to inquire about his workout plans for the day. Manish used to train bodybuilders across Delhi and was a competitive weightlifter himself until recently. While his own body continued to remind others of these past achievements, it also made no secret of the fact that he himself was no longer 'in the game'—he had clearly been in better shape. He combined management of the gym with a number of other enterprises he was in the process of developing, such as a gym in Dwarka near the airport, and one at a company at an industrial site nearby. Manish was a fitness entrepreneur, and the effort he put in to maintain his body was mainly about showing his clients that he knew what he was talking about.

## DIVERGENT BUT INTERSECTING TRAJECTORIES

Supriya, Amit, Sunil, Manish, Ratish and Ravi could be found at BodyHolics most mornings. For an hour or more they would occupy the same space, breathe the same air, watch the same Bollywood videos and interact with each other. Outside the gym, however, their lives were highly divergent. Amit and Manish were from Chirag Dilli, and still referred to themselves as middle class with some hesitation. Supriya, Sunil and Ratish, who lived in colonies adjacent to the gym, could be considered upper middle class.

Ravi stood out in this group. He grew up in GK-II as the scion of a family heavily invested in construction projects across the National Capital Region. Never his ambition to join the family business, Ravi opted for a career in fitness training instead. In roughly half a year with BodyHolics, he had emerged as one of the leading figures on the gym floor, providing coaching to the other floor trainers, assisting Manish with his plans to expand his fitness business, and providing training to a select number of clients, including me.

Even if it is hard to determine the actual size of the Indian middle class and its various subsections, on the gym floor, middle-class hierarchies were always perfectly understood. With the exception of Ravi, the two groups—trainers and clients—could be divided neatly along lower and upper-middle-class lines. At the same time, boundaries and demarcations were constantly explored, tested and, depending on whom I asked, trespassed as well. Within the context of the gym, a certain social and cultural flexibility appeared possible that one also found in outlets of Starbucks and in high-end malls. For those pursuing upward social mobility, these spaces seemingly encouraged disobedience towards adhering to how middle-class belonging was interpreted elsewhere.

In terms of economics, fitness training was hardly ever the most lucrative route to follow, though. Starting salaries for floor trainers were as low as Rs 8,000, making it barely more profitable than being employed as a security guard or driving a taxi. Yet, unlike such professions, salaries tend to increase quickly once a trainer manages to bring in personal-training clients. While Amit was not making much more than a starting salary, Kishore from Chembur made ten-fold that amount as a personal trainer to clients in the upmarket areas of Mumbai.

Over coffee one afternoon in a bakery near the gym, Ravi tells me his impressions of the backgrounds and ambitions of various floor trainers at the gym. As a fitness trainer of an upper-middle-class background, he was well-aware of his in-between, somewhat liminal, position. He often functioned as a go-to person and translator of sorts for the trainers, not so much in terms of language—almost all trainers and members of the gym were native Hindi speakers—but with respect to expectations and comportment.

Ravi thought of his fitness career as catering to various ambitions. On the one hand was his desire to make it big in fitness because of his 'sound knowledge of different techniques', most of which he had picked up by studying various websites and watching YouTube videos. On the other was the even bigger ambition of making it as an actor. Although a north Indian by birth and upbringing, he had his eyes set on Kollywood, shorthand for the Tamil movie industry located in Kodambakkam, Chennai. He was particularly invested in exploring a connection with Kavya, a female client who was one of the morning's regulars and who could often be found in his company. A freshly graduated doctor, Kavya had recently joined a practice in nearby Saket, but her father apparently had links with the movie industry in their native Tamil Nadu. Ravi was never short of dreams to share in this regard. When he was not practising his rudimentary Tamil with Kavya between workout sessions, Ravi could be found in the company of Manish, who had eagerly involved him in various plans to expand his fitness business, relying on Ravi's superior grasp of the English language as well as contacts and background.

Quickly gobbling down a few sandwiches the afternoon we met for coffee, Ravi started by pointing out that the main difference between him and the other trainers was his capacity to speak English. For Amit and Kareem, the latter a trainer with whom I did not interact much, 'speaking English is like climbing Mount Everest barefoot without an oxygen mask'. Manish, on the other hand, simply needed to boost his confidence, Ravi assured me. His English was much better than he himself thought it was. Some of the spot boys who came in irregularly did not speak any English at all. It was hardly necessary, since their main task was to put the weights back after clients were finished with them.

Yet, Ravi thought it crucial to invest in their English-language capabilities as well since much of the information about fitness training online was in fact in English, and it would be 'the only way to grow in this business'. Besides that, clients appeared to appreciate it when knowledge of various fitness techniques was conveyed in English.

The strength of BodyHolics as opposed to other gyms, in his opinion, was the sense of family which the gym strongly encouraged. 'We are all friends, we work like that accordingly.' Although most gyms appeared to revolve around and stimulate similar notions of family and camaraderie, Ravi was adamant that there was always unwanted competition in other gyms, with trainers trying to steal each other's clients, because of the commission received for personal training and the status associated with having a large client pool.

BodyHolics had a better model, Ravi argued, providing on-the-spot personal training without charging clients extra for this service. It was all part of the package, as was the vision. Within this context, each trainer had his own strength, which the gym utilised to full advantage. 'I see the client's personality and then I give them the best trainer.'

Kareem was known for his 'chocolatey eyes' and his 'easy relationship with the ladies', while Amit was appreciated for being a 'hard worker who brings out the best in clients'. The two were childhood friends from Chirag Dilli and had joined around the same time. Girish, a lanky, agile senior trainer, originally from the state of Odisha, was particularly appreciated for his patience and his knowledge of different workout techniques, yoga among them. His backstory was something of a mystery, with rumours about a wife and possibly kids back home in a small fishing village. Then there was the one female trainer, Mishty, who doubled as a receptionist and occasionally provided aerobics classes.

Any trainer, however, should be able to take over if a colleague is absent, Ravi emphasised. Trainers' frequent absences were due not only to illness or family obligations, but also because of the high rate of attrition. Ravi could not say why so many trainers quit, but it was likely the low pay that BodyHolics offered and the absence of personal-training opportunities, as well as the frequent gossip about the gym's financial state and its general state of neglect.

## RAVI'S DOWNWARD MOBILITY

Ravi completed his schooling at an all-boys English-medium school, after which he graduated from Delhi University's College of Arts and Commerce. Although he had subsequently enrolled in a master's course in counselling psychology, Ravi felt he was not in the right place, not least because after a couple of months, he already found himself 'teaching the other students'. He had little interest in joining the family business, but there was considerable pressure on him to give up what the family thought of as an idle pursuit that would never generate the kind of income that the business would. The idea of working on building sites and 'having to talk with the labourers all the time' was simply not something that appealed to Ravi though. Mainly employing semi-skilled and illiterate Bihari labourers, it would require him to 'to use very rude language, otherwise they won't listen'. To this, he added: 'You can't talk to them in any other way. You have to use shit language.'

There was something else: 'I want to be self-made.' Ravi stated with confidence: 'I can sweep a floor, I can build a wall,

I can do all that.' Of one thing he was certain, though: 'I want to do something on my own without anyone's help.' He added almost defiantly: 'I never wanted to go down the line that I got my father's help.' It was one of the reasons he did not get along with his father too well at the time. 'My father and I, we are not that close right now. We don't talk much at all.' His father thought that, unlike his brother, Ravi was not 'strong enough' and that that was why he did not want to join the family business. 'I did have that dream to be an architect when I was a kid. Unfortunately, I did not have that science much under control, I was not very good at it.' He had even 'prepared' for his civil service exam, but it had also not proven to be his calling. 'I wanted to … I wanted to do well but I never really wanted a desk job per se.'

Finishing a chocolate roll and flushing it down with a can of Sprite, Ravi asked me if I had seen the 2004 movie *Swades*, starring Shah Rukh Khan. The storyline resonated with his own, he felt. In *Swades*, the protagonist, on leave from his job with NASA, returns to India where he becomes involved in a project to solve the electricity issues of a small town. The idea appealed to Ravi at a social as well as personal level. Having told his father that he would not join the family business, he needed to find an alternative to prove that he could be successful in something else. 'That's when I started working out. I wanted to put all that energy into something and that's where I could put it in.' It was really something he could put his heart and soul in, he found.

As a way of developing and educating himself, Ravi started looking into the biomechanics of fitness, and realised 'how it worked and how I could improve it'. Determined to find the best workout possible, he was able to transform his body within four months, Ravi said with great pride. 'I went from being a matchstick to being a real man. To a man's body!' He suggested he was 'almost anorexic before that' and overtly self-conscious of this. From this moment, he became 'truly devoted to fitness'. It was now his 'number one ambition' to feature on the cover of the Indian edition of *Men's Health* one day. But Manish, his boss and friend, had warned him that he first needed to 'complete a certain fitness level'. In terms of natural good looks, he was already there, Manish said, but for the magazine to take him seriously, he would have to work on his body and come up with an innovative workout routine that he could pitch.

Parallel to these plans was Ravi's desire to make it as an actor. Movies had played a significant role all his life, he said. 'I come from a family where Bollywood is praised to a level that there is a television in our home which only shows movies.' (He meant that there was one movie DVD or the other playing almost all day.) However, he was not very fond of cinema as a kid. 'Unconsciously it was projected on me.' Searching for the right way to phrase it, he clarifies that 'unconsciously I was getting the movie stuff'. He used to see himself as a beta character, 'never this alpha guy that I am now'. Bollywood functioned as a prime source of inspiration—'I always wanted to be this superhero guy'—but his shy character stood in the way.

As a young child, Ravi would spend considerable time watching movies with his grandfather. Reflecting on his younger self, he suggests that 'unconsciously you watch this a lot, and that's how I imagined myself to be an actor'. In his spare time, he had developed an interest in books that combined philosophy and psychology. He declared proudly that he had a knack for emotions and that he was quite good at reading them. Fantasising about himself as an actor, he emphasised that he wanted to give it his best shot. 'I want to have that emotion.' By this he meant being able to evoke an emotional reaction from the audience.

Ravi was working hard on his Tamil because Kavya might be able to get him a role in a production. He dedicated forty-five minutes a day to it, quite a challenge given the hours he had to put in at BodyHolics. 'I give myself self-affirmation. I tell myself that I am good in Tamil, am fluent in Tamil.'

## Manish's Upward Mobility

Manish was a veteran in the field of fitness compared to Ravi. When I first met him, he was twenty-nine years old and a personal trainer with various certifications—from aerobics and weightlifting to those with a focus on the needs of professional athletes—and even experience in physiotherapy. He was also a registered pharmacist and dietician. Before he made his move into fitness, his main passion was wrestling. 'I used to do that at a state and national level.' This was not kushti, which is practised in local akharas[72] but 'the wrestling they do at the Olympics'. That said, Manish had also been involved in traditional wrestling for about five years. It was the most exhausting thing he had ever done, he once said. He still had some friends who competed in various akharas, but he had lost interest in it a long time ago. Manish saw no future in the sport, and even noted that some of the akharas he had once trained at had now been converted into gyms, some even with air-conditioning.

In the morning, we often found ourselves in his small office, which was located in the middle of the gym. Through the tinted windows, he could keep an eye on what was happening on the floor. There was even a little bell to summon people to his office or for the music to be changed, though the latter was often so loud that the bell could not be heard and Manish had to dash out of his office to deliver instructions in person. In contrast to some of his floor trainers, Manish preferred that Western music be played, since BodyHolics was 'a high-class gym' and he would 'get complaints' if it played Bollywood music non-stop.

He described BodyHolics as 'high class' as if oblivious to the desperate state of some of the equipment, which was a source of amusement among the regulars. The gym's financial predicaments were well known, and some clients wondered openly if Manish would be able to pay the electricity bill in time so the air-conditioning could be switched on in the hotter months. However, its strategic location in GK-II and its mainly upper-middle-class clientele added a certain élan to the place— to Manish at least. His friendship with Ravi mirrored this, in that he considered him crucial to the future of the gym. Ravi's upper-middle-class upbringing would certainly help in his expansion plans and add high-end clientele to the gym, he reasoned.

Usually comfortably seated behind his desk, Manish had at least two phones in front of him, one for business, the other for personal calls. On the wall behind him was a large image of the goddess Kali, as worshipped in the nearby Kalkaji mandir. On the other hung a somewhat kitschy affair of a couple of horses in flight, galloping to some unknown destination. It was the kind of image one could buy by the dozen not far from the gym, outside Nehru Place metro station at footpath stalls.

Although Manish described his family as lower or new middle class and mainly educated in Hindi, he would also say they were 'a family of business owners, engineers, doctors', and never failed to add that nobody was doing what he was doing. His parents really only thought of 'two fields that way'. One either became an engineer or a doctor, other ways of making money were never quite considered. 'They think more about earnings, not what the child wants, the child's happiness.'

Although he could never get himself very interested in the field of medicine, he did complete his pharmacy certification and was employed with a large pharmaceutical company for a while. 'But I was not enjoying it over there. I even got the offer to work in Dubai, Saudi, Singapore.' The thought of working abroad was attractive, but the work itself did not hold enough appeal.

'I like instructing people ... I like it when students listen to me and take my advice.' This is also why he got along so well with Ravi. 'He really treats me like a teacher.' Although BodyHolics was closed on Sundays, in the afternoon he would invite all the trainers to the gym to provide additional coaching. 'I also have this anatomy book from which I teach them.' It was the kind of foundational knowledge that they could also get from a certification course with Gold's Gym Academy or elsewhere, but he had little faith in the quality of such training institutes. 'On Sunday, I teach them about fitness, client scheduling, slow knowledge, things like that.' He feels he has a similar student–teacher relationship with the bodybuilders he had taken under his wing in order to prepare them for regional and even international competitions. One of the bodybuilders he was involved in coaching at the time was sponsored through the Central Reserve Police Force. As Manish explained: 'He will not do any job there, he just takes a designation, that's all.' They also did not really have the capacity to work in the police force, he found, at least not at the level they were getting paid for. 'They are just focused on their sports, those guys.' Also, 'They come from humble families, they require this money to survive in their sports.'

Although Manish described his own origins also as humble, he took a superior position when compared to the bodybuilders he trained—not just as their coach or guru but also in terms of his middle-classness. Even if he frequently voiced doubts about his ability to speak 'proper' English, compared to them, he was a man of the world, well connected in the world of business and sports. At the same time, he noted that there was a wide gap between his own position and that of his gym's clients. Such discussions always oscillated between how impressed Manish was with the clients he got to interact with, and the respect he would receive from them.

One morning, when he and I were hanging out in his office and discussing future plans for the gym, he suddenly pointed at a woman doing leg-extensions and asked me if I knew what she did for a living. I had spoken to her a few times, but this had never come up. 'She is a CMO with Vodafone, she heads the marketing department there.' He leaned backwards, his hands behind his neck, and stared at the ceiling for a while, then suddenly exclaimed: 'She calls me sir!' To emphasise the significance of this, he added: 'That makes me feel high, it makes my level feel high. In here, they call me sir …' Illustrating how exceptional her calling him sir was, he added proudly: 'Outside, I would have to make an appointment.' While he was signifying that he was only a nobody, unlikely to have such acquaintances or connections, it became clear that his familiarity with her was clearly very much bound to the gym itself.

Only with very few clients did he have a relationship outside the gym as well, though it always appeared as if this was still very much in a preliminary stage. A client with whom he hoped to develop a further relationship was a local business owner who had recently opened a shopping mall nearby. Such people held a specific interest because they might facilitate the opening of another gym in the future. Whenever this client came in, Manish would greet him warmly and make sure that he personally provided the training. Often, I could hear them chat about their respective businesses, exchanging ideas and suggestions in a mixture of English and Hindi. From the body language, it was also clear that the relationship was not that of equals. Manish, however, never failed to emphasise how much he 'learned from that guy, especially about doing business'. This idea of learning from his clients was constantly on his mind, and although he avowed a fierce passion for fitness and helping his clients lose weight, gain muscles and become healthier in general, being in the gym was also an opportunity to extend his contacts, work on his English, share business ideas and, more generally, learn from those he held in high esteem.

Throughout our conversations, questions about how Manish came across in terms of speaking English, his comportment and sense of style, his presentation skills, even the car he drove frequently came up. It would be a mistake to think of him as insecure though. He was perfectly at ease with who he was, where he came from and what he had accomplished. It was only that, when it came to his clients and the lifestyle he sought to emulate, he realised that there was a gap he had not yet successfully been able to bridge. Particularly revealing were his excursions outside the gym in order to meet personal clients at their homes, for which he would bring Ravi along. Not so much to help him with the training, but to guide him in terms of how to deal with such clients. Manish framed it as an opportunity for Ravi to learn, but it was also clearly an opportunity to educate himself. Among these clients he counted a dealer of luxury cars, a number of property developers and various other businessmen. 'These are sophisticated people, so we have to behave ourselves.' Some of them even had a gym-space at home. Pondering on this some more, he offered: 'We have to know how to behave around them. These are high-class people; it is good to get exposed to them.'

## A Departure from the Gym and Life

I returned to BodyHolics after a brief absence in early 2014 to find that things had changed dramatically. Ravi had inexplicably left BodyHolics and joined his father's company, seemingly having given in to family pressure. He was not speaking to anyone, Manish and others assured me, and there was no point contacting him. According to Kavya, he was not interested in meeting anyone from the gym, and he was 'mainly keeping to himself' after he had left. She had visited him at his home and had also spoken with his mother, but had returned home without a clear picture of what was going on. Apparently, she had even been able to secure a small role for him in a Tamil production through her father. 'But he said he wasn't ready.' It had surprised her, considering how enthusiastic he had been before. However, looking back on the weeks before he had stopped coming to the gym, there had already been something off about him. 'Something was clearly on his mind but he was no longer sharing it with us,' Kavya said.

One evening, a few weeks later, Supriya contacted me by message to ask if I had heard 'about Ravi'. My immediate reaction was one of excitement, thinking he may have re-joined the gym, but there was something ominous about her messaging me this way. Watching her 'typing a message', I suddenly dreaded the worst. Ravi had indeed taken his own life.

In the week after, the gym remained quiet. Clients seemed to think most trainers would not show up for work, or that the atmosphere would not be conducive to working out. Those who did visit the gym put little effort into their exercises, instead congregating in the centre of the gym to exchange ideas, theories and rumours, keen to understand why Ravi had committed suicide. Such conversations invariably turned to the question of choice itself. As one regular customer, a rather striking senior woman usually dressed in all-black, a number of large diamond-encrusted rings adorning her fingers, put it: 'He was such a gentle soul, he really wanted to do something else in life.' She had known the family for years, lived in the same neighbourhood and had occasionally tried talking to him, she said. He had always treated her with a generous amount of respect, she remembered sadly. Her sentiments resonated with that of the other women who had been regulars most mornings.

Ravi's suicide had brought people together, but their sadness could also be framed as a performance. All agreed how unfortunate it was the way things had turned out, yet their accounts and reasonings were also laced with a certain sense of understanding. The general consensus was that family pressure, the desire to do something different and the relatively little space he had to manoeuvre had left Ravi with no other choice. This was also not the first suicide they had dealt with in their circle, nor would it be the last, it seemed.

For Ravi's family, working in the gym signified a form of downward socioeconomic mobility that they had not been able to stomach. Not only would he not be able to make the kind of money the family business promised to generate, he would end up serving customers that the family considered their equals. This contrasted with the way Ravi perceived the situation, considering his career in fitness as an alternative that had great potential. It was a firm belief he shared with Manish, who despite his different socioeconomic background, had also faced backlash from his family for the choices he had made.

## STARTING A NEW GYM, A NEW LIFE

During the third week of February 2014, Manish invited me along to an industrial estate owned by a global provider of telecommunication solutions. He had learnt that they wanted to open an in-house gym and he was hoping to become the manager. The day before, we had discussed his plans at a Starbucks in Nehru Place, going through his PowerPoint presentation and thinking of possible questions they might have. He was keen to bring me along, partly because he thought a 'foreign face' would help smoothen the deal—providing the plan with cosmopolitan élan, so to speak—but also because he felt that his English was not strong enough, even though the conversation was likely to be in Hindi.

He would have brought Ravi along for a meeting of this sort, but now Manish had to rethink some of his business plans. The mere mention of Ravi usually brought tears to his eyes, and in the last one-and-a-half months since his suicide, Manish had repeatedly recounted how the family had called him to take care of Ravi's body when they found it lifeless in his bedroom.

Over time, Manish had begun to involve me in his plans to expand his fitness business, seeking my advice over how to formulate a 'proper email' in English or to read through a folder he had prepared. In the past, Ravi had been part of these plans. Together they had visited nearby housing societies in order to pitch fitness-related ideas to the inhabitants. In these upper-middle-class compounds, Ravi had been crucial in introducing him to the people in charge, because they required an introduction from a trusted face. Manish explained: 'We try to meet their residents and give them some coaching and counselling.' He hoped they would join BodyHolics, but his staff could also offer training at the housing society, if desired.

'A lot of them have sitting jobs, they sit behind the computer, they are not fit, so we tell them the benefits of working out. What the importance of the workout is.' As always, he would bring along a slide-show to convince his audience of this. 'We give them a piece of paper on which they can write three questions.' He would take these questions into account to make them a group offer, or if it was a company, a corporate deal. In some cases, he had been lucky and managed to sign on new clients, but often they were met with disinterest and prejudice. 'They have a lot of doubts, these people, lot of questions.' Bringing Ravi along was by no means a guarantee of success. 'They will want to know why he is there, what is he doing in fitness.' Yet, with Ravi at his side, Manish had felt much more confident. In the car, on our way to the company site, he repeated how much he missed Ravi when he made such visits. Admittedly, he wasn't making that many. 'I lack the motivation for it.'

The number of clients at BodyHolics had reduced drastically now that Ravi was no longer around. As such, Manish really needed this new gym to 'work out'. 'It's like Ravi took the soul out of the gym with him,' he remarked, pensively staring at the traffic that was snaking past at a snail's pace across a flyover. As always, the trainers were changing on a regular basis. Girish had absconded to Odisha to take care of family matters, and it was unclear when, if ever, he would be back. Animosity was also brewing between Amit and Kareem, who were no longer on speaking terms because of a conflict that appeared to revolve around a female client who was possibly married. Kareem had been providing her with 'personal training' at home, something Amit did not approve of, or was jealous about.

Manish wanted to lay-off Kareem 'because his enthusiasm for the work is gone'. Abounding rumours over the alleged affair also had to be considered. These were the topics Manish and I had discussed at the Nehru Place coffee shop: departing trainers, concerns over declining gym memberships, clients demanding the return of prepaid fees and the cost of starting a new gym. Besides, there were always the nagging doubts about how those Manish considered higher-up would perceive him. Would his English be sufficient? 'We never spoke that language at home, Michael.'[73] Would they even hear him out? 'I am not from that world, man,' he once said, pensively.

On his first visit to Starbucks, I could see he was uneasy, even though he was familiar with the brand. The chain's ambitious plan of expansion across the city fascinated and bewildered him. Dressed neatly in branded jeans, a T-shirt which fit perfectly and accentuated his powerful build, with multiple smartphones resting casually on the table in front, Manish was evidently ill at ease, commenting that this was hardly his usual place to meet people. He explained that this was typically a place where he expected 'hi-fi people' ('like you') to hang out. At the same time, he seemed eager to thank me for suggesting this location, seeing it as an opportunity to learn more about what was going on in this world that he aspired to belong to one day.

While going through his presentation, Manish appeared edgy about pitching this idea of an in-company gym. He remarked that this was something he had imagined Ravi would have done for him, or at least to have helped him with. He had consulted some BodyHolics' members, including a former client who was working 'somewhere high up in a telecom company' and who had looked at a few of his PowerPoint presentations before. 'She makes 1.5 lakhs [per month] but is doing this to help me,' he explained. That way, he put considerable faith in the socio-cultural capital of other people (including me, a firang pursuing a mystifying research topic), even though he himself was clearly the expert in fitness and bodybuilding. Although Manish's English had improved over time, certainly since I had first met him, he continued to lack confidence, mainly because of the way he interpreted his own vernacular upbringing in relation to those he hoped to convince of his expertise and knowhow. Ironically, 'life coaching' was becoming integral to the way he had started pitching his fitness ideas to companies and housing societies lately. One of the exercises he liked to introduce at company outings had a team-building element to it: he divided a team into three groups and gave them each a rope and wood to cross an imaginary river ('this was really good fun'). He was all about problem-solving, he assured me, and since he had overcome considerable obstacles himself, he was the perfect man for the job.

During the thirteenth-day memorial service, the local Arya Samaj temple was packed. Around ten regular clients were there, as well as fellow trainers such as Girish. Absent, however, was Amit, who had shown considerable anger about Ravi's suicide. 'He would always show his positive side here but he was negative inside,' Amit had blurted out. Ravi had been like a brother to him, he felt. 'He always gave me proper respect!' The fact that Ravi had taken him seriously and had invested time helping him improve his skills, even becoming a friend of sorts, were memories he now cherished. Knowing how much resistance Ravi had received from his family, he felt justified in not attending the memorial service, as a form of protest. Manish understood Amit's point of view but felt compelled to attend anyway. The family could have known that Ravi was depressed and 'should never have allowed this to happen', Manish said, though.

In our interactions, either in the gym or in the car going somewhere, Manish would frequently complain of how little support he received from his family. 'They don't believe in this at all, they don't know what it is.' His brother, who was employed as an engineer, was especially negative. 'But he's just jealous, that guy,' he had said once, dismissively. The second-hand car he had recently bought was deemed 'too high' for his family, as he put it himself. 'They think I am wasting my time, that I am taking too many risks.' While he admitted that they have a reason to be worried, since his fitness business was not doing so well, he also felt he needed the car to 'show people that I am doing well, you know'. Having made our way across the flyover, nearing the site where he envisioned his next fitness business would take shape, Manish repeated that he felt he was on the way to something big. But like the traffic we had just been in, he knew that the road ahead was congested, and that he was not nearly close to where he wanted to be.

## The Possibility of Alternatives

Earlier in this chapter, I described Amit and Supriya watching a song from *Goliyon Ki Raasleela Ram-Leela*, a film which revolves around a Romeo and Juliet-type fable, represented by the impossible love between the son and a daughter of two warring clans involved in the local arms trade. Both Amit and Supriya agreed that Ranveer was looking incredibly fit; however,

Supriya added that she fiercely disliked the 'loudness' of the character the actor depicted. She had seen the movie in its first weekend and had even attended some promotional event related to it at nearby Nehru Place, but wished she hadn't. What she found particularly disturbing was the amount of sex and violence portrayed. She wasn't the only one who found the movie problematic. The intended title of the movie had caused controversy prior to its release. Its initial title, *Ram Leela*, had been attacked by various groups that were angry the film's 'vulgarity' was being connected to the story of Lord Ram. As a result, the movie had been renamed *Goliyon Ki Rasleela Ram-Leela*[74] only forty-eight hours ahead of its release.

In the movie, the hero and heroine commit suicide in the end, something that ultimately brings the two warring clans together to cremate the bodies of the young lovers. At BodyHolics, Ravi's departure not only brought two 'opposite' middle-class groups together, but also made them (temporarily) reflect on their position vis-à-vis each other. Here, perhaps, was it laid out in the clearest manner how social and cultural mobility in urban India produces a complex interplay of overlapping, intersecting and occasionally contradictory trajectories. I knew Ravi only briefly, and even though we became quite close during that period, I am sure there are aspects of his life that he did not share, experiences that I was not aware of, and that what he provided me with was an edited version of a story he 'liked' to share. It was by no means an easy decision to write about this incredibly bright and caring trainer whose untimely departure from the gym and life affected and impacted a whole range of people. Yet his story is too important not to share, not least because it shows how difficult it can be to choose an alternative career trajectory and 'to do things' differently in a new India.

CHAPTER 3

# BODY | BUILDING | CAPITAL

*'Each workout is like a brick in a building, and every time*
*you go in there and do a half-ass workout, you're not*
*laying a brick down. Somebody else is.'*

– Dorian Yates,
Mr Olympia Winner, 1992–97

This Monday morning, Express Avenue, one of Chennai's premier malls, is reasonably quiet. Victor sits in front of me, his heavy arms resting comfortably on the table, a tray with a large portion of French fries, a double Whopper chicken and a sizeable Coke waiting for him. Although the plan was to meet for coffee, Victor was hungry and in the mood for 'some decent food'.

Just two days earlier, Victor had made his return to the bodybuilding stage at the third Mr Steel Tamil Nadu competition after a long absence due to a back injury. As we get ready to dig into our hamburgers, he seems to be in a much better mood than at the competition, where he had taken third place in his particular weight category. Smirking, he says, referring to the bodybuilder who had placed second: 'That guy had no legs!' He quickly takes a bite of his burger and continues: 'See, he was very broad in his chest and shoulders but he had no legs, so I should have beat him on this.' Apparently, the jury does not like Victor, a problem I have heard him complain about before. 'I could see it from their eyes, when I started posing they all stopped smiling and looked down.'

He believes one of the jury members—a bodybuilder who was once Victor's training partner, but with whom he had since fallen out—is the culprit. Victor thinks he had instructed the other jury members to place him lower than he actually deserved. 'I used to respect him quite a bit in the old days. I really thought that he is a genius, that guy.' This memory triggers a diatribe about several other bodybuilders who all work as personal trainers and who apparently 'show many different faces' depending on the situation they are in. 'Online they will be like, don't take drugs, they're bad for you, but in the gym, they are the big guys who will supply you with anything they can get their hands on.' There is a lot of back-stabbing and jealousy, he explains. 'They don't like me because I am an IT guy. They think I am only doing it as a hobby and that I don't need to win.' The competition came with a generous cash prize which the jury may have thought to be of little consequence to him. He has now decided to change bodybuilding federations for good. 'This federation is not showing me any respect and will never let me win.'

When I had reached the competition at Kamarajar Hall in Teynampet, Chennai, two days earlier, the first categories, from 55 to 70 kg, had already taken the stage. An energetic host had asked for the audience's special attention for the upcoming category of men with various disabilities, such as a missing leg or an underdeveloped body-part due to childhood polio.

A raucous applause greeted the competitors, who all received a certificate of appreciation for their participation. Next was the 70-plus category. Around ten gold-painted men started nervously flexing their leg muscles, encouraged by the droning voice of one of the jury members who instructed them on what pose to take and what muscle group to flex next. Some were dressed in professional posing trunks, others were simply wearing underwear smudged with the tanning lotion they had lathered on. It was as if a giant had picked up each of these men by their heads, holding them between index finger and thumb, and dipped them in gold paint. The untanned faces took on a ghoulish hue under the harsh stage light, with chins jutting through paper-thin skin and eyes lying hollow in their sockets, the result of extreme dieting and dehydration.

In India, bodybuilding competitions usually commence with the lowest weight-category of 55+ kg, after which they work their way up by increments of 5 kg. Since the 100-plus category is the highest one, this means that there are roughly ten different weight categories in all. The winners of each category compete for the overall title in the final round. Considering the muscular size and maturity required to win an overall title, it is usually awarded to one of the winners of the 80-plus to 90-plus categories. In comparison with the lower-weight categories, these bodybuilders are able to display larger and more detailed body-frames and vascularity. Besides that, their muscles tend to have reached a particular maturity that comes with years of working-out. The higher weight categories often have an issue with fat levels and dryness, which stands in the way of giving the muscles a particular definition and veiny-ness.

Other categories, such as the disabilities one, or those that revolve around fitness or swimwear modelling, are sometimes added to give the competition an extra dimension. Depending on the location, sponsors and federation involved, there are also specific moments scheduled to honour the local organisation, the owner of the building or the land at which the competition takes place, and the senior bodybuilders present in the audience. These men are asked to flex their muscles for the benefit and appreciation of the audience. Bodybuilding competitions in India, therefore, rarely run shorter than four hours, though double that is no exception. As one informant jokingly put it: 'It's like a day match,' referencing cricket, India's national obsession.

## Bodies Building Capital

In the third Mr Steel Tamil Nadu competition, Victor competed in the 80-plus category and hoped to have a chance at the overall title. The winner's prize was well-deserved, and Victor had stood no chance against him. However, it was up for debate whether Victor should have come in second. Having made considerable investments in his physique in terms of time, energy and money, it was thus not surprising that he had left the competition feeling disillusioned. What drives bodybuilders to invest inordinate amounts of time, energy, not to mention actual financial capital into their bodies? What are their bodies ultimately about? Is it mainly a quest to become huge, something that is imbued with notions of masculinity, in order to impress and dominate through sheer physical presence? This last question is mostly rhetorical, as indeed, these bodies stand for much more than hastily drawn conclusions about gender and sexuality. The personal histories of the bodybuilders I met and interviewed across India showed that the process of 'building bodies' is intimately connected with strategies of upward mobility, middle-class belonging and, ultimately, a changing Indian economic, social and cultural landscape.

The focus in this chapter is on men whose bodies are considerably larger and more muscular than those featured on the cover of the Indian edition of *Men's Health* and other male-oriented lifestyle magazines, or those that film stars build their storylines around. Finding a balance between the body required to be competitive on the bodybuilding stage and the lean, muscular ideal foregrounded in popular media doesn't necessarily entail a physical process per se. Instead, capitalising on the bodybuilder's body requires a translation in terms of what clients may potentially read in it. In order to better appreciate what is at stake here, I focus first on the long-term trajectory of Victor, a Tamil bodybuilder from a Brahmin family and a former IT professional with a multinational company in Chennai. His case makes for an intriguing comparison with that of Akash, a bodybuilder with international ambitions who lives and works in Bangalore, India's IT heart. Like Victor, Akash is competitive on stage as well as a successful personal trainer. However, unlike Victor, who pursued running his own gym after quitting his IT job, Akash is employed as a highly sought-after personal trainer with Gold's Gym.

Their bodies are not the product of a mere strict adherence to highly specific diets and routines, but of an intimate understanding of what they are doing. While their bodies might provide the impetus for clients to seek out their services, it is ultimately their knowledge of how their bodies can be transformed that makes Victor and Akash successful and sought-after as trainers. Another instance of capitalising on this knowledge is that of Kaizzad Capadia (actual name), a former bodybuilder who now runs a training institute offering certification courses to aspiring fitness trainers—something leading fitness brands such as Gold's Gym and Reebok are also involved with. The success of Capadia's training programme shows that 'training' trainers has become a source of income in itself. Ultimately, the question I shall investigate here is not only what it takes to build a muscular body but also what is required to capitalise on this body.

## INVESTING CAPITAL IN THE BODY

As the overall category was taking the stage at the end of the competition, I sat next to the parents of the eventual Mr Steel Man 2017. Dressed in a colourful sari, the winner's mother was lost in prayers. The smell of the jasmine flowers in her hair mingled with that of the protein powder added copiously to water bottles around me, as well as the lingering odour of the 'coconut-flavoured' tanning lotion of the bodybuilders who had already competed.

During an earlier posing session, I had been drawn into a conversation with some male students sitting next to me. They said they were avid gym-goers but had no particular desire to compete themselves. In fact, none of them looked particularly muscular, and they assured me that their interest was mainly in the spectacle that was unfolding on stage. They had heard about the competition via the gym they attended, and decided to attend since they had no other plans for that particular Saturday evening. Throughout, discussing the various candidates on stage, they remained ambivalent about what they were actually observing. They were decidedly proud that Tamil men could display such muscularity, but did not quite desire this for themselves. One of the men, in the process of finishing his degree in accounting, professed: 'That's not for us, really. We're just students, just having a good time.'

Attending a newly established private business university on the outskirts of town, they were from Chennai and would occasionally attend bodybuilding competitions 'such as this one'. Familiar with Bollywood movies, they were, however, quick to turn the conversation to Kollywood, underlining that their superstars were 'into fitness as well'. They asked me if I was familiar with Surya, Atharvaa or Prabhas, the last primarily a Telugu actor. Prabhas's performance in the first part of *Baahubali* (2015) had showcased his incredibly muscular physique. As soon as Prabhas became the main topic of conversation, others joined as well, and declared their admiration for one of the key moments in the movie when the actor, playing the character of Shivudu, carries a huge Shiva lingam out of the river, on his massively muscular shoulders.

There was indeed something about the sheer might and charm of the character of Shivudu (or Baahubali), portrayed by Prabhas with undeniable vigour and humour. At the time, the second part of the movie had yet to be released, but part one continued to enchant masses across India. Looking at the stage and watching the competitors in the overall weight category, it was clear that one of the attractions of attending this competition was to see men 'like Baahubali' flex their muscles, posing to the rambunctious applause and whistling of those in attendance. However, for Victor, this had been a very serious occasion, far removed from the world of Tollywood or Kollywood; he was returning to the stage after years of absence. A back injury had prevented him from competing earlier, but equally, prior disappointments, disillusionment and even depression had stood in the way of finding his way back into the limelight. Now he was about to show how his form had improved, how his knowledge of various training techniques had benefited him, and ultimately, how his detractors and competitors had been wrong all along.

Discussing what it took for him to get competition-ready as he finishes the remainder of his Burger King meal, Victor provides a rather blunt calculation of the costs involved. Over a period of five months, he estimates he has spent around Rs 70,000, nearly one month's salary, to get where he needed to be. This included money spent on whey-protein powders, metabolism enhancers/fat burners, various other supplements such as L-Carnitine, glutamine, amino-acids and vitamins, daily doses of chicken and eggs (about thirty egg-whites per day), vegetables for the necessary fibre, fish twice a week, and costs related to body-enhancing drugs, as well as medicine necessary to flush the liver and kidneys afterwards. These costs were certainly not exceptional. Bodybuilders across India had provided me with similar summaries, in certain cases even estimating that they had spent as much as Rs 30,000 per month for a period of up to half a year in order to become competition-ready. In Victor's case, the money necessary for this had come out of his own pocket, working as a team manager with PayPal, but other bodybuilders I had gathered data on over time had relied on a combination of income through personal training and support from family or friends.

## A BODYBUILDER'S CAPITAL INVESTMENT

A bodybuilder's body represents capital, not only in terms of what has been put in it but also what can be capitalised on.

As much as the two seem to speak to each other, they can be decidedly at odds as well. The concept of bodily capital, which initially emerged out of Pierre Bourdieu's (1978) writing, provides some helpful tools to understand what the issue is here. While the concept has regularly returned in social scientific explorations—often in relation to the energy, money and time people invest in their bodies—it remains a rather elusive concept that heavily draws upon symbolic interpretations. As such, the male body's capital can be equated to its approximation of a particular masculine ideal, signalling potential attraction and eliciting desire. It aligns with hegemonic notions of masculinity: raw power, steadfastness, discipline and control, and the potential of domination over other men.

Loïc Wacquant (1995), writing on the practice of boxing, presents a somewhat deviating view, highlighting a universe in which the body is primarily understood as an asset, an instrument and object of work.[75] In this perspective, personal bodily worth becomes a product of accumulated labour. Through this lens, we can understand boxers as entrepreneurs of bodily capital.[76] If we follow this line of thought, we see how the gym can be thought of as the factory space that converts bodily capital into pugilistic capital, able to deliver the sharp upper cut, the powerful lower cut and ultimately the deafening knockout to win a fight. This is what evokes applause and appreciation from the audience. The notion of muscular armour is particularly relevant here: the product of intense training and workouts, it makes the actual fight possible.

Parallels can be drawn between the boxer and bodybuilder's bodies in the way they get shaped and moulded in the gym, and eventually in how they take on the identity of a fighter who can defeat his competition on stage. But in the world of bodybuilding, it is not just the immediate reward of winning a competition that matters, but also what the body communicates when the spotlights are off. A bodybuilder's physical capital is thus not necessarily something that only matters during a competition. In the Indian context, one could argue that winning competitions is only peripheral to 'building' the body. Prize money tends to be low and the cost of preparing exorbitant. Besides, the various titles on offer are of little value due to the many different federations involved, and the limited recognition and appreciation contestants receive from the public at large. Bodybuilders who can sustain themselves on prize money alone, or whose annual prize money even approximates the money invested in becoming competition-ready, are extremely rare. Titles won—whether Mr India or Mr Karnataka or Mr Coimbatore—are not only referred to on bodybuilders' social media profiles to underline accomplishments and successes, but most of all function as a way to emphasise their knowledge of bodybuilding itself. What these men display on stage is not just an outer shell of rock-hard muscles and garden hose-sized veins, but also a transformation imbued with notions of physical labour, dedication and having made the right choices with respect to workout routines, diets and the use of supplements and other substances. Their bodily capital is thus the sum of being as well as becoming a bodybuilder.

Bodily capital exists alongside economic, social and cultural capital, yet it is also deeply entangled with these other forms. In the case of India, it can be employed or utilised to compensate for the lack of other kinds of 'capital', but this requires a negotiation of sorts. While it can be employed to close a perceived gap in middle-classness, it's not an easy matter of add and replace. In the first chapter, Kishore and Vijay utilised their bodily capital to strategise a path to upward mobility, and in a sense Manish, Amit and their colleagues at BodyHolics of chapter two were doing the same, building on their expertise to make a living as well as climbing the middle-class ladder. However, none of these men were bodybuilders, nor did they aspire to be. Kishore sometimes participated in MuscleMania[77] competitions, but he would compete in the swimwear or modelling categories, where the globalised standards of competitive bodybuilding do not apply. In fact, he was always deeply ambivalent about the sport of bodybuilding, which he equated with risky health decisions and bodies that did not appeal to his client-base.

So what parameters guide the idea of the 'ideal type' of muscular body? The bodybuilder's bodies that Victor and Akash sport are decidedly bigger, more muscular and vascular than those idealised in Indian cinema. In fact, if such a body makes an appearance in Indian movies, it tends to be one that references aggression, violence and, to a certain extent, 'stupidity'. In the Telugu action movie *Srimanthudu* (2015), which narrates the story of Harsha Vardhan, a young man who inherits his father's business empire, this is precisely what happens. Knowing little of his father's background, Harsha starts exploring his roots and ends up in a remote village in Telangana's hinterland, which he subsequently adopts. This angers a local crime boss, and ultimately leads to a showdown from which Harsha emerges victorious.

Actor Mahesh Babu, who plays the lead, is not known for his shirtless scenes or muscularity, unlike his brother-in-law, actor Sudheer Babu, who has made his 'transformed' body part of the way he promotes himself. However, in this particular movie, the character Mahesh Babu portrays is endowed with incredible strength and a fighter's capabilities. Taking on the village strongman's posse, consisting mainly of bodybuilders, the contrast is easily made between Mahesh Babu's lean and athletic body and that of the bodybuilders he takes on one by one, without breaking a sweat. Only two years earlier, in 2013, the actor had made a formal announcement that he was working on his six-pack abs, which had promptly led to fans photoshopping his body with those future abs. These photoshopped pictures, which can still be found on the internet, also show that this imagined future did not have Babu looking like the henchmen he takes on. Yet, despite this 'popular' depiction of the bodybuilder's body—as equated with underworld or goonda figures, and thus with aggression, violence and other uncouth behaviour—there is still something that allows competitive bodybuilders like Victor and Akash to attract clients of upper-middle-class backgrounds. How do bodybuilders and their clients negotiate the difference between the lean, muscular bodily ideal and that which is required for a bodybuilding competition? To understand the complexity involved, a deeper examination of bodybuilding in India is needed, in terms of its practice, organisation, history and ultimately what matters when on and off the stage.

## What the Bodybuilder's Body Stands For

In the West, the practice of bodybuilding has long been associated with the working-classes, perhaps because of the easily drawn parallels with physical labour.[78] Such interpretations are layered with a particular normativity that locates the 'pursuit of bigness' within a class-based context. It is perhaps no surprise that bodybuilding has frequently been thought of as 'masculinity run amok, a frightening example of alienated behaviour, or a disturbing expression of narcissism'.[79] Alan M. Klein's landmark study *Little Big Men*, which came out in 1993 and focused on one of the best-known gyms on the West Coast of the United States, stands out. Zooming in on the gendered aspect of bodybuilding, Klein explores this in relation to issues of health, sexuality and the willingness to push the 'spatial' boundaries of the body. Klein's study is particularly revealing for its study of the economic aspects of bodybuilding and the impossibility of combining this pursuit with a more ordinary existence.

Lee F. Monaghan's *Bodybuilding, Drugs and Risk* (2001) builds on Klein's assertion and focuses more explicitly on risk-taking behaviour, the use of drugs (anabolic steroids, growth hormones, etc.) and the idea of the perfect (bodybuilder's) body. While such studies have greatly contributed to a deeper understanding of bodybuilding in a Western context, they do perpetuate certain commonly held notions and assumptions about the sport's location within class hierarchies, its problematic relationship with masculinity, and how this body is assumed to be the product of the copious use of steroids and other harmful substances.

Bodybuilders like Victor are aware of such ideas and deeply critical of them. To them, such concepts reduce their bodies to failed ones: freakish make-believe bodies that could not, or should not, have a place in reality. These ideas rest too on the contradiction represented by the strength of muscles versus the weakness of mind of a person who has succumbed to the use of illegal substances to grow in size. It does not take much to think of the lean, muscular body with its 'natural' assumptions of fitness and athleticism as the healthy counterpart, one that popular culture has not only rendered acceptable but, more importantly, also desirable. Mobilising bodily capital through a narrative of transformation offers bodybuilders like Victor a way out of this predicament, centering their know-how. Even if a bodybuilder in question has pushed the physical boundaries of his own body beyond what a client might desire for himself, the notion that transformation is possible still appeals.

Interviews as well as casual conversations with bodybuilders across India revealed that they thought of their bodies as works of art, though principally in unfinished terms and as works-in-progress. Their employment of the term 'sculpting', with the gym providing the tools, contrasts markedly with the kind of 'working-class' lingo used on the gym floor in order to describe attempts towards transformation. Victor emphasised the 'hard physical labour' that went into his body; during a competition in Delhi, bodybuilders described it as requiring 'heavy lifting' and 'back-breaking work'; and in Mumbai a personal trainer and MuscleMania participant referred to a session that had gone particularly well as 'killing it'. It was generally agreed that it had to hurt for it to work, and that pain was one's best friend. One should leave the gym feeling depleted, having turned on 'beast mode' so as to 'destroy the body'. Like factory workers at the end of a long day, they envisioned themselves going home exhausted but satisfied with a job well done and another day put in.

Sociologist Pamela L. Moore (1997) argues that built bodies can be understood as 'the ultimate expression of the postmodern belief in corporeal malleability'.[80] Such bodies are almost absurdly controlled, as Moore puts it, the flesh really no longer flesh, the body having become a machine, 'as when builders describe their arms as guns or their legs as pistons'.[81] The practice of bodybuilding thus resonates with what is expected of working-class sports such as boxing and rugby, which revolve around pain and suffering as well as gambling with the body.

Evidently, this contrasts with a middle-class interpretation of the body as an end unto itself, as well as for others to view, admire or appreciate.[82] Yet as anthropologist Niko Besnier (2012) also points out, the relationship between sport and class designations is historically as well as spatially unstable.[83] Class dichotomies, therefore, mainly serve as a tool, not a rule.

There is something paradoxical about the fact that, while the bodybuilder's body is seen as the product of hard work and heavy lifting, signalling a working-class background, it was also bodybuilding that gave birth to the emergence of the fitness industry and eventually produced a new middle-class bodily ideal.

While in the West, the new bodily ideal has generally led to a demise in the popularity of bodybuilding as a competitive sport, with gyms divorcing themselves from any association with bodybuilding altogether, in India, bodybuilding competitions have gained in popularity. This is not as contradictory as it first appears. While, elsewhere, fitness has gradually come to replace bodybuilding and its associated aesthetics, in India, the two are umbilically linked through the narrative of transformation, which resonates with the way 'new India' itself is constantly under construction.

The idea of the malleability of the body, of possible mastery over it, is an important one. In a fast-changing society where nothing appears stable and solid, knowing which direction to head, what choices to make and how to regain or retain some form of control lies at the heart of what trainers as well as their clients seek. This was also what *Men's Health* offered; the magazine did not simply report on the latest workout techniques for reducing weight and 'building muscles fast', but simultaneously layered this with notions of cosmopolitanism, success and ultimately being in control and being able to withstand the caprices of rampant consumerism.[84] While bodybuilders may 'embody' this information, being masters of their own bodies, developments in the sport itself seem to reflect the haphazardness and speed of urban India's transformation. Their lives are precarious and uncertain. On an individual level, this is reflected in the high costs and low earnings that the sport entails, while on a more general level, this precariousness reverberates in the organisation of the sport itself with its multiple associations, federations, competitions as well as business people and politicians involved.

## THE ANATOMY OF A SPORT

The evident rise in popularity of bodybuilding as a sport is handicapped by two developments. First, the rapid proliferation of competitions held at town, city, state and national levels, often making use of similar titles, such as Mr Delhi, Mr Haryana, Mr India and Mr South Asia. Besides, the associations and federations involved frequently change their names; old ones merge and new ones emerge. When I once asked Victor to provide me with an overview of the various competitions in which he and his students[85] had participated in 2017, these included, other than the one already mentioned, the Mr Tamil Nadu Amateur competition, the Open State meet (held in the town of Thiruchendur), as well as various other competitions, such as the Senior Nationals IBBF, the State Powerlifting Meet, the Open State Meet and so on. Another well-known Tamil bodybuilder, who now runs a popular gym in Chennai, provided a radically different list. Some of the men he trained had participated in a Mr Chennai competition, while others had joined the stage in something called the NABBA Mr Tamil Nadu,[86] the Open Single Category State Championship and the Mr South India Contest.

A brief survey of the Delhi–NCR region provided an equally dizzying array of competitions and titles. A young bodybuilder from the state of Haryana reported that he had recently won in his specific weight class of 65 kg in the following competitions: Mr Delhi, Mr Haryana, Mr North India and Mr India. A Rohtak-based bodybuilder mentioned he had participated in Mr NABBA India (in Gurgaon), Mr Haryana and Mr Himachal. However, the Mr Haryana he competed in was not the same as the one mentioned earlier.

Newspaper reports of 2017 show a similar picture in other parts of India. Goa held a 'Federation Cup National Bodybuilding & Physique Sports Championship' in the city of Margao in May; the town of Shajpur in Madhya Pradesh held a 'divisional-level bodybuilding championship' in December, and that same month, Punjab's industrial city of Ludhiana hosted the Mr Libra 2017 competition, while the city had also played host to the Mr North Zone competition three months earlier. In early 2014, I was able to attend no less than three different Mr Delhi competitions in the course of only ten days, all organised by different Delhi-based associations, held in locations that were mere kilometres from each other.

A piece in the *Shillong Times* by one Bhattacharjee from Guwahati, who claims to have been involved in bodybuilding for thirty-five years, underlines this complexity.[87] Reacting to an earlier news report[88] about Meghalaya bodybuilder and cop Prosonto Basumatary's alleged participation in what the author mistakenly refers to as 'Mr Universe Body Building Championship' (the actual name was Mr Universe Championships) to be held in Budapest, the writer is principally bothered by the involvement of the Meghalaya Body Building and Fitness Association (MBBFA), which accordingly is affiliated to something called the World Amateur Body Building Association (WABBA). As the author claims: 'The Indian Body Builders Federation with its headquarters at Mumbai is the only federation recognised by the Government of India, Ministry of Sports and Youth Affairs.' He continues that this is the only body which can send participants to international competitions. He is sure that there is no Mr Universe competition in which India is taking part. What amazes him even more is that the bodybuilder in question is 'not even a zonal champion, far less a national championship[89] (in his weight category)'. What follows is an allegation one regularly comes across while discussing the state of bodybuilding in India with competitors, jury members and others involved. '[M]any unauthorised and dubious organisations are springing up and to justify their existence promoting sub-standard body builders who are winning "high sounding titles," and getting undeserved temporary publicity.' What the author appears to find particularly problematic is that the bodybuilders involved are 'short-circuiting hard-scientific workout and becoming BIG by random use of banned drugs'. Accordingly, the state of Assam itself has three different Mr Universe competitions which 'faded away from public memory within weeks'.

In 2015, there were at least three associations involved in organising various competitions ranging from Mr Chennai, Mr Tamil Nadu and Mr India in Chennai. By 2017, this number had grown to six, each with their own competitions. It was a pattern that kept repeating over time. The involvement of official and unofficial federations and associations—often helmed by men who had business interests in the sport (for instance, as suppliers of protein powders or gym equipment), or who played a role in local politics—meant that the field was constantly in motion. With this proliferation of competitions and organisations came added pressure to be relevant and to imbue the promised titles with a certain gravity in order to be taken seriously. As a result, increasingly, well-known American bodybuilders, who have competed in competitions such as Mr Olympia (Joe Weider's Olympia and Fitness & Performance Weekend) and Mr Universe (Universe Championships) are lured to India as special guests at events, or to be part of new gym openings to imbue them with additional prestige. Seven times winner of the Mr Olympia title, Phil Heath, four-time winner Jay Cutler and Ronnie Coleman—considered by many as the greatest bodybuilder of all time, with eight straight wins at Mr Olympia—have all visited India in recent years. Making use of the opportunity, (aspiring) Indian bodybuilders go through great lengths to meet their idols, proudly shaking hands with them and posting pictures of the occasion online.

American bodybuilders come to India not just for the generally 'handsome'—though rarely disclosed—fees offered for appearing at the event. They also charge for signature and picture events, score endorsement deals with whey-protein powder and supplement brands, as well as use the opportunity to spread the word about their own online-coaching services. Clearly, for 'celebrity' bodybuilders from the US, India's rapidly expanding bodybuilding scene offers interesting business opportunities that may be lacking at home.

## THE HISTORICAL BODY

The visits of well-known US-based bodybuilders, whose posters adorn gyms across India and often feature prominently on local bodybuilders' Facebook walls as a source of inspiration, hark back to the Indian tour that 'strongman' Eugen Sandow made a century ago. Visiting the cities of Bombay, Calcutta and Madras between 1904–1905, he apparently whipped up a 'physical culture craze'.[90] Between 1900 and 1907, Sandow was the most famous strongman on the planet, and considered to be the world's strongest, most beautiful man, even an apostle of physical culture.[91] Not unlike current-day fitness celebrities, such as Simeon Panda or Lazar Angelov,[92] Sandow claimed to have over a million followers around the world as early as 1904.[93]

Carey Watt, who conducted extensive research on Sandow's India tour, argues that he was already well-known in India years before he arrived.[94] His visit sparked phenomenal interest in his system and products, and inspired men to not only build muscles but even to grow Sandow-like moustaches. Sandow's popularity across the globe emerged out of a momentum that had been gaining steam for a while already. As Dutch sociologist Ruud Stokvis writes, 'From the mid-nineteenth century onwards, self-styled strongmen began to appear throughout Europe and the USA.'[95] Thus, Sandow was far from the only one who could count on a considerable following and popularity. Referred to as 'physical culturalists' at the time, there was the 'Danish Apollo' Jørgen Peter Müller, Britain's Eustace Miles, the American Bernarr Macfadden, France's Edmond Desbonnet, and even India's own Kodi Ramamurthy Naidu.[96] The emergence of a so-called Körperkultur in German between 1890 and 1930 was particularly influential in propelling the popularity of strongmen and working out among men in countries such as England, France and the US.[97] The 'philosophical' muscular Christianity movement that had its origins in England in the mid-nineteenth century also played an instrumental role, with its focus on strengthening, building and maintaining the male body. Notions of patriotism and masculinity were layered with notions of athleticism, fitness, beauty, discipline and even sacrifice.[98]

Born in East Prussia in 1867, Sandow started out as a wrestler who occasionally supported himself as an artist's model until he won his first strongman contest in London in 1889. At the time, 'physical culture' consisted of a combination of what were deemed rational and scientific approaches to improving one's health and fitness, usually combining an amalgamation of calisthenics, gymnastics, weightlifting and breathing exercises.[99] Unlike current-day bodybuilding, Sandow's focus was less on building or showing muscles, and more on teaching 'the gospel of health'.[100] It is this focus on health that characterises the contemporary fitness movement, and also what has gradually eroded its direct relationship with bodybuilding.

Sandow considered his India tour 'something in the nature of a triumphal procession'. He was mightily pleased with the successes he had booked with his 'treatments' as he called them, and reported that the 'natives' had found them to be 'almost miraculous'. In Sandow's Magazine, he went on to belittle Indians, even recycling Lord Macaulay's disparaging assertion that Hindus were the children of children, and were 'weak even to the point of effeminacy'.[101] Sandow was clearly influenced by a Western way of thinking about the 'oriental other', which in India rendered certain groups or castes as incapable, inferior and feminine. While Jats, Gurkhas and Rajputs were celebrated for their military prowess and fighting capabilities, other Hindus were thought of as categorically weak.[102] Such demeaning colonial characterisations eventually also contributed to the lift-off of India's own involvement in fitness.[103]

Irrespective of Sandow's impact, towards the end of the nineteenth century, there was a burgeoning fitness movement in India that reached its zenith in the 1920s.[104] Anthropologist Joseph Alter notes various influential figures, such as Kodi Ramamurthy Naidu, who developed a scheme of mass drill exercises; Baroda-based Rajratan Manikrao, who established gymnasiums that adopted a type of paramilitary drill regime; and the Raja of Aundh, who made surya namaskar exercises popular. Around this time, the game of kabaddi was routinised, the YMCA developed a way to train physical education instructors and yoga was reinvented. Under the leadership of Hanuman Vyayam Prasarak Mandal, Indian athletes toured Europe in the 1930s and went on to demonstrate various Indian gymnastic routines in the Lingiad, an international physical culture competition in Sweden. Furthermore, a number of publications that provided an overview of India's history and involvement with gymnastics and athletics saw the light of day, hammering home the point that India had a long-standing connection with quests for male health and fitness. Joseph Alter argues that:

> As such it was a clear statement against the pervasive colonial idea—or sense that there was an idea—that India was a country made up of listless, sedentary peasants, reclusive otherworldly ascetics, overfed Brahmin priests preoccupied with scholarly learning, and ruthless, pernicious despots ... [105]

## CASTE AND MIDDLE-CLASS HIERARCHIES

Recuperating the Hindu masculine self remains a concern for Hindutva-oriented organisations, and is occasionally touched upon in scholarship and documentaries that discuss, though often only peripherally, the connection between bodybuilding and local politics in India.[106] While it is true that a well-known bodybuilder such as Suhas Khamkar has occasionally flexed his muscles in the company of politicians—for instance with the Shiv Sena chief, the late Bal Thackeray[107]—such connections are invariably more complex than the picture conveys. Khamkar, a Central Railway employee, is partly sponsored through the so-called sports quota that enables talented athletes like himself to take up government positions. It is thus not surprising to see bodybuilders associate with politicians and government officials if the occasion arises. There is a clear dependency. Jury members of bodybuilding competitions, and those involved in associations and federations, also act as gatekeepers of eligibility for these sports quotas, potentially able to facilitate (or deny) coveted 'symbolic' positions with the railways, police force, army and so on. At competitions, this is generally cause for considerable suspicion and gossip, especially when it seems that another bodybuilder should have been awarded first place instead. While I have always understood such discussions to relate to a deep-seated sense of bodily insecurity and even inferiority that almost all bodybuilders I met over the years carried with them—causing them to constantly discuss and report on their 'haters', 'backstabbers' and 'small men who don't matter'—the monetary dimension of this resentment should not be disregarded. A sports quota job guarantees a steady income and the freedom to truly invest in one's bodybuilding career.

The connection between politics, Hinduism and bodybuilding is a complex one. This is just as true for caste. The popular association of the sport with rowdy or uncouth behaviour—the goonda figure and the brusque doorman—is often followed by the all-too-easy conclusion that these must be men of lower or at most intermediate caste backgrounds. When I discuss my work with fellow academics, they tend to assume that these must be Jat or Gujjar men. These 'easy' associations point to an understanding of middle-classness which is still undeniably governed by the implicit idea of an internal hierarchy. It is in such assumptions that we also find a particularly puzzling aspect of what class actually denotes in India. If we take middle-classness as a social and cultural construct that is centred on relative positions, its assumed relation with particular caste groups has a tendency to equate upper-middle-class identities as those 'truly' belonging to the middle class. It renders the rest as newcomers, or worse, pretenders.

## A TamBrahm Body

The first time Victor provided me with a glimpse into his personal biography was on a Thursday afternoon in September 2015. I had made my way to Karappakam, an enclave situated between the IT hubs of Thoraipakkam and Sholingallur, home to multiple multinational companies such as Accenture, Capgemini, Infosys and Tata Consultancy Services. Meeting me over lunch at his company's canteen, housed in a tall glass-fronted building, Victor was dressed like any corporate professional: a short-sleeved button-down shirt, neatly pressed pantaloons and a pair of decently polished though somewhat dusty leather shoes. It was quite a different look from what he usually displayed to his fans online: either a tight-fitting T-shirt of some sports brand, or simply his underwear.

Seated at one of the long tables in the canteen, about to delve into a sizeable plate of vegetable biryani, it was hard not to notice how Victor's body evoked a sense of discomfort. Casual glances from canteen staff and colleagues confirmed what he had told me earlier, that his muscles always triggered a rather convoluted mixture of admiration, fear and shock. 'Right now I am normal, but when I am eating my veins start popping out. People get grossed out by that.'

Victor had not always looked like this. 'I started thin but then I became a fat teenager,' he told me. Born and brought up in an impoverished Tamil Brahmin household in Chennai, Victor described his childhood home as one of the few with an actual roof in a slum-like neighbourhood. Having worked for a cable company when he was younger, Victor's father met with an accident and was unfairly terminated. He subsequently established a typewriting institute but struggled with deteriorating eyesight, only to eventually go blind altogether. His father used to be 'quite fit and muscular himself', and in fact, 'used to work out often', Victor recalls fondly. It is to this that he traces his initial fascination with 'getting big and strong'. An incident in his childhood left a particularly strong impression on him. Victor was playing outside with his brothers when a cow suddenly charged at them, and his father managed to stop it by grabbing it by its horns.

Even more influential, however, was finding a poster of Dorian Yates, a former Mr Olympia who had gone on to win six consecutive titles between 1992 and 1997. Victor saw the poster on his way home from school, in a second-hand bookstore that eventually provided him with some initial bodybuilding literature, and the image never left him. To date, he has that image on his cell phone. Although he was enthralled by Dorian Yates's massively muscular body—'He even seemed to have muscles on his feet!'—Victor quickly realised that he did not have the 'proper genetics'.

He needed to fuel his body with proteins to bulk up, but in his Brahmin vegetarian household, there was an injunction against cooking meat at home. As a solution, he installed an electric kettle in the backyard, but could only use it when his mother was not washing or drying clothes. Moreover, he was always worried that his Brahmin neighbours would complain about the smell of meat being cooked. Later, it was a bit of an issue in office as well. Desperate to increase his size, Victor knew the vegetarian canteen wouldn't do, and so resorted to other means of getting his proteins in. 'I would bring these tins of tuna to work but couldn't eat them at my desk.' The smell would bother his colleagues, many from Brahmin and vegetarian households themselves. 'Instead, I would go on the fire escape and eat it there.' He would make sure to brush his teeth afterwards.

Although Victor's mother is now proud of his accomplishments, she was not happy when he broke the news to her that he wanted to 'get into bodybuilding'. Initially, she thought he was 'into stripping or something', and needed extensive convincing, not to mention his father who, even though he was a muscular youngster himself, could not imagine what this path would lead to. Yet, the family was hardly a stranger to making 'alternative' decisions to facilitate upward economic and social mobility. Although he grew up in a 'very proper TamBrahm household', Victor had been enrolled in a Hindi-medium school. His father hoped this would provide him with the necessary set of skills to make his way into a respectable government job, for which Hindi would not just come in handy but would simply be required. His father claimed to have experienced considerable discrimination in his own career for 'not being able to speak proper Hindi' and had wanted to prevent his son from experiencing the same thing. As a result, Victor never learned to properly read or write Tamil. When as a teenager he became a regular contributor to the Tamil-language bodybuilding magazine that was sold at the second-hand bookshop where he discovered Dorian Yates, this was an obstacle from the onset. So, he wrote the articles in English and his mother would translate them into Tamil.

The first gym Victor joined at fifteen was not really a gym, as he puts it himself, 'more like a floor with no roof and just some odd dumbbells'. At the time, he paid Rs 30 per month, a sum which sounds pitifully small now but still had him carefully considering if his pocket money would cover it. From this neighbourhood gym, he moved up to a gym that was attached to the college he had joined, and which was charging Rs 100 per month. This one did have a roof, but as it was located in a basement and did not have any windows; it was dark, stuffy and quite hot. It was only at the third gym that Victor seriously started thinking of becoming a bodybuilder himself. By that time, he had started taking advice from a senior collegemate who had won some competitions and who had made an impression on him. Doing research on the best way to grow his muscles, he quickly realised that no one he knew would be able to give him 'the right information'. All this changed when he met Arasu Mounaguru, 'the biggest Indian I had ever seen'. At the time, Arasu ran a gym called Gold Gym,[108] a non-aircon kind of a place, geared primarily to youngsters who aspired to become bodybuilders. Arasu continues to be an influential member of Tamil Nadu's bodybuilding community, running several gym chains and being a judge at competitions held across the state.

## A Body of Information (Technology)

Victor showed me around his office, taking me to the company gym that he occasionally used for his own workouts. Still dealing with a back injury, he was focusing mainly on cardio-related exercises as well as his arms. He already sported massive eighteen-inch arms, but had long been fixated on this part of his body and believed that they could get even bigger. When I met him two years later at the Mr Steel competition, he proudly informed me that they were now twenty inches, though he had had to give up a full inch to get his body 'dry' enough to become competition-ready. He looked ready to take on his rivals, phenomenally muscular and exhibiting a fighter's glare I had not seen for a while. His arms were seriously 'the guns' he had envisioned. That same year, Victor also participated in the annual Mr Tamil Nadu Bodybuilding Championship. The locality of Palavakkam where it is held is not the immediate surroundings one might associate with such a competition. As an article in the *The Hindu*[109] put it: 'known for its bustling adjoint IT parks and traffic, [Palavakkam] is also known for its increasing love for bodybuilding'. The general secretary of the Tamil Nadu Body Building Association, R.L. Thiruvengadam, said succinctly: 'You must be here to believe it.' Around one thousand men, women and children came to witness the event. The Palavakkam area sports around twenty gyms of which no less than ten are specifically geared towards bodybuilding.

There is something inherently odd about a bodybuilding competition taking place in an area predominantly housing

IT companies. It is not only the connection to information technology and thus something that utilises the brain more than the body that feels aberrant here, but also the association with what is regarded as a typically upper caste, and even Brahminical, type of profession that is characterised by studying and, most of all, mathematics. Yet Victor, an IT professional as well as Brahmin himself, was deeply immersed in bodybuilding even before he had ever set foot in any one of these IT offices. Although he combined his IT career with providing online coaching to aspiring fitness enthusiasts and other bodybuilders, his day-to-day expenses were essentially met by his earlier investment in his engineering degree, which had provided him with his first job in an IT company. Eventually, he quit his job with PayPal, and took on personal training as a full-time profession, earning an average salary of more than Rs 1 lakh per month.

Growing up in a lower-middle-class (though decidedly upper-caste) milieu, and receiving most of his schooling in English and Hindi, Victor now makes more in his 'new middle-class' profession than he did in his 'typically' upper-middle-class (and upper-caste) profession as an IT professional. While his switch from developing software to providing personal training could be construed as downward mobility in social and middle-class terms, he has made this shift work in a way that justifies the initial gamble. However, for him to be able to embark on this journey, he had to convince his parents and wife who were worried he was giving up on a stable income in a job that came with promising career prospects. At a certain level, the two professions were not altogether that different, he argued. Both relied heavily on knowledge, on knowing and understanding how things work, whether a computer system or the body. While bodybuilding does not immediately evoke an association with learning or studying, bodybuilders across India underline their 'knowledge' as crucial to success in the sport as well as to generate an income out of personal training. What personal-training clients eventually seek to understand is how to transform their own bodies and what it requires in terms of workout routines, diets and supplements. This, in its most concrete form, is the capital that the bodybuilder's body represents. Investing in the body and building it till it is competition-ready signifies an understanding of how a body works and what can be accomplished with it. Those successful in the business of personal training, which not all bodybuilders necessarily are, exude the confidence that the transformation of their own person can also be replicated in another's.

Akash is a Bangalore-based bodybuilder whose aim is to become internationally competitive. Unlike Victor, who now runs his own personal-training business, Akash is employed by an international gym chain, for which he works on a commission basis besides receiving a baseline salary. The city of Bangalore is well known as India's IT capital and for its relatively large proportion of highly educated urban professionals. Some fifteen years earlier, when I was researching the emerging IT industry in India, Bangalore was the one place where gyms were already commonplace and easily accessible. Influenced by management styles that originated in Silicon Valley and which piggybacked to Bangalore when transnational IT companies such as Texas Instruments, IBM and Oracle started establishing themselves in the city, most office buildings and campuses were quickly outfitted with well-equipped gyms.

Like other Indian megacities, Bangalore now sports gyms in almost every locality. Akash is a relative newcomer to the city, attracted by Bangalore's economic prospects and assumed quality of life. While he did not move to the city to become a bodybuilder or personal trainer, it was the direction his career would eventually take.

## BUILDING A BODY IN INDIA'S IT CAPITAL

Akash enters the restaurant we had arranged to meet at on 100 Feet Road in Indiranagar, one of the city's most upmarket areas for shopping and retail, with a helmet under his arm. He excuses himself for being late, and makes a casual reference to Bangalore's increasingly worse traffic situation. The arrival of the IT industry is generally held responsible for this, having robbed the former Garden City of its trees, the Pensioner's Paradise of its calm and the (naturally) Airconditioned City of its cool. Long-term residents of Bangalore, whether Kannadiga or not, regularly lament the demise of all that once made Bangalore such an attractive 'middle-class' city with its beautifully kept bungalows, neatly trimmed lawns, and the need for sweaters in the cooler months. Today, Indiranagar has gradually come to epitomise its enduring identification as India's Pub City, with multiple craft breweries, cocktail bars and lounges flanking both sides of 100 Feet Road. But, until recently, this was a quiet inner-city neighbourhood with a mainly upper-middle-class population. Indiranagar's transformation into a leisure district has brought with it considerable infrastructural concerns, which the area, as the rest of the city, seems unable to adequately deal with.

Urban scholar John C. Stallmeyer discusses Indiranagar in his book *Building Bangalore: Architecture and Urban*

*Transformation in India's Silicon Valley* (2011) and notes how initially the area was intended as a residential quarter for the city's growing population. Even though most of its infrastructure was in place by 1983, it would take till the end of the 1980s for many of the building sites to reach completion. Now considered decidedly inner-city, until the 1980s, the area was thought to be too far from the heart of Bangalore. To Stallmeyer, Indiranagar represents a 'patchwork of urban fabrics', home to industrial and government complexes such as Hindustan Aeronautics Limited (HAL), the Indian Space Research Organisation and the National Aerospace Lab. The area therefore hosts part of the knowledge industry that gave impetus to and facilitated the rise of the city's IT industry. Yet, now it doubles as a prime destination for upper-middle-class professionals, eating at boutique-style restaurants, shopping at designer furniture stores and drinking craft beers. This is true of other areas in Bangalore as well. In 2003, auto drivers would generally refuse to take passengers from the city centre to HSR Layout where I stayed at the time, a locality beyond Koramangala with a relatively easy commute to Electronics City, home to, among others, the headquarters of Wipro. In 2019, it is a sought-after enclave with its own shopping malls, fast-food restaurants and booming property market. There is no shortage of gyms in the area either.

Akash, who grew up in a family he describes as 'a little less than middle class', regularly makes his way to Indiranagar to hang out with 'friends' or to meet clients who might be interested in hiring him as a personal trainer. His family, originally from Darjeeling, moved to Calcutta, where Akash grew up. He moved to Bangalore about a decade ago, in search of a job in order to take care of his ageing mother. Although providing fitness training was already on his mind, he initially made a living selling encyclopaedias door-to-door, and as a call-centre employee with a local company. Now employed as a personal trainer at Gold's Gym in Richmond Town, an upper-middle-class locality that traces its origins back to 1883, during British rule, Akash makes around Rs 70,000 per month, considerably more than the Rs 7,000–8,000 he made in his early days as a floor trainer. He gets Rs 10,000 per personal client per month, coaching them thrice a week. What the client pays per month to Gold's Gym is considerably higher, of course. Like most gyms, Gold's Gym works with a commission-based structure, and trainers double as salespeople who need to make sure they bring in the necessary clients.

Akash claims to be unsure if he has ever made the required target, and even seems unaware whether he is a silver, gold or platinum trainer, designations that the gym employs to reflect seniority, certifications obtained and other markers of distinction. This status also corresponds with the rate that the gym charges for personal training services rendered. Akash says it all matters very little. He is never short of attention in the gym and, as he puts it, 'always keen to help others'. While his body stands out in any situation—such as in this restaurant, where the waiters can barely conceal their glances as they prepare our coffees—his fluency in English and his general ease with clients makes him particularly popular among high-end members. Among them are a fashion designer from Miami who, at fifty-five, 'still has a very good body', and an obese five-foot-tall female manager who has decreased her weight from 89 to 68 kg with Akash's help. It is these results that matter, he stresses, 'this is also what people see in the gym'. He means that it is not just his body that gets noticed, but what he manages to do with others' bodies as well.

While part of Akash's income goes to his mother, a widow who lost her husband, a police officer, a number of years ago, his main expense is the maintenance and preparation of his body for competitions. One day he hopes to hold an IFBB[110] pro-card, but already there are some international competitions on the immediate horizon that he wants to participate in if he can find the necessary sponsor. In order to become competitive internationally, he has taken two online courses with professional bodybuilders in the US. For a complete course of around five months, such bodybuilders charge an average of Rs 3 lakh, about four months' worth of Akash's salary. 'I was only able to afford one month really, but I did learn a lot of new techniques that way.' When he is preparing for an important bodybuilding competition, Akash spends around Rs 70,000–80,000 on his body, which does not even include the growth hormones that he cannot afford for now. Even if his body is central to his sport and the main vehicle for earning an income, it is 'the feeling of being pumped, the tightness setting in' that is his chief motivator. 'That's the addiction,' he says. For a more recent competition, he had trained three times a day and lost 28 kg over a five-week period. 'I really pushed my body to the limit that way.' He had to be really disciplined to achieve this goal. 'No salt, no carbs or even water towards the competition.'

Akash has been able to supplement his income with some occasional modelling; for instance, he recently did a photoshoot for a new protein brand that was being launched in India. 'But it's not my world,' he says. 'People are too fake'— something he had also noticed on a recent trip to Mumbai to participate in the MuscleMania competition being held there. Attending a gym near the venue for a last-minute workout, he had noticed 'the looks and stares' he was receiving. 'A lot celebs train there.' Apparently, actor Salman Khan's brother had spotted him and wanted to talk to him. 'He had asked his own trainer, "who is that guy?"' But Akash claims he had been too shy to talk to him. Just by being in that gym, he realised that he could 'make quite a bit of money there if he moved to Mumbai'. However, Bangalore has become his home, and he is unsure if he would be able to provide training to the more elite clients he met in Mumbai. When he was in Kolkata recently, he had overheard a trainer and his client talk about him in Bengali, which they assumed he did not speak, discussing the shirt he was wearing and saying something like 'that must be a rich guy'. The shirt was a gift from a client, an aspiring actor, but the association made him sad, knowing his own 'humble background' and what others read in his body and demeanour. The client in question later prepared for MuscleMania himself. Akash says, 'He hopes to win and then increase his fan following online.' Apparently, 'he thinks that that will get him noticed and finally get him into a movie'. But there is something inherently sad about the client's efforts, Akash feels. 'Sometimes I think: get a life man, you're always on the phone, you are not living.' Reflecting on the popularity of working out and building muscular bodies, he says: 'Being on stage for show-off fuels it now, but it's hard to maintain such a body.' It's something he knows all too well.

Akash's body represents considerable capital, most obviously in terms of what he has invested in it over the years—copious amounts of anabolic steroids, growth hormones and less 'problematic' supplements. Fluent in English due to his convent education, he bridges the gap in middle-classness rather easily, even if he is constantly aware of how he navigates the socioeconomic space that separates him from his clients.

Photos on social media narrate his journey from an 'average Joe' to a muscular hulk, and help convince prospective clients by demonstrating how extensive his own transformation has been. Yet, Akash's bodybuilding ambitions go well beyond what he has achieved so far, and the money he makes through personal training is not nearly enough to cover the cost of 'getting bigger' as well as continuing to support his family. While he is hopeful a sponsor may knock on his door one of these days, his predicament typifies the burden and limitations of bodily transformation.

## Selling the Future Body

Located in Santacruz East, a municipality of Mumbai not too far from Bandra West, K11 is a training institute that specialises in offering certification courses to aspiring fitness trainers. Its founder, Kaizzad Capadia, is a well-known senior bodybuilder, and can often be found giving guest lectures at fitness and bodybuilding events. One such event, Sheru Classic, was held in Pune in 2014. I arrived early to secure a seat; the room was bound to fill up, considering its limited capacity. While waiting for Kaizzad to take the stage, I entered into a conversation with Sunny, an enormous six-foot-plus tall Sikh Punjabi who was living in Mumbai and worked as a pilot for one of the budget carriers. He wanted 'to become huge, that's why I am here', to which he added with a smirk: 'I want to become bigger than Kaizzad.' Sunny had started bodybuilding in 2009 when he was still stationed in Kolkata, saying that the main inspiration had come from a colleague who was 'pretty big'. His father was a chief manager safety with an aviation company himself. 'I was born into a flying family is what you could say.' Having completed his training in the Philippines with a bottom-end training school ('There were lots of accidents, like one plane could not get its wheels down, one coach and two students died in a crash.'), it is now his income as a pilot that funds his ambition 'to become truly huge'.

We discussed the 'huge' aspect further while we waited for Kaizzad to arrive. 'I eat thirty eggs a day, the egg yolks as well.' According to Sunny, it was just a myth that you should only eat the whites. 'I learnt everything from Kaizzad. His stuff is just damn amazing.' He regularly checks Kaizzad's blog and the K11 website. 'I follow all of that now.' Employing Kaizzad's 'wisdom' allowed him to increase his weight from a skinny 75 to 105 kg at some point. However, Sunny then had to lose weight for his job. 'You're this eight-pack but they don't care about that!' Since the standard uniform no longer fits him, he has it stitched near his home in Powai. It is worth it, though, Sunny said. His parents were initially apprehensive about him taking 'all these proteins and pills', but when they started seeing results, they were impressed. Although he was not doing any steroids at the time we met, he was 'definitely contemplating them' for the future.

A huge round of applause erupted when Kaizzad finally took the stage, followed by some whistling and cheering. When the audience had calmed down, Kaizzad came straight to the point. The central question he wanted to address that day was how one can increase one's muscles when one does not have the strength. The audience seemed confused. Behind Kaizzad was a contraption that allowed for various exercises. Keen to break the gender balance, Kaizzad invited some 'tiny girls' onstage 'to lift some weights and do some squats'. Joking about the industry's obsession with certifiable and proven techniques, he added that what he suggested was 'a scientific way', one he followed himself. At the same time, he stressed: 'There's a right way and a wrong way. But there is no Kaizzad way. There is only the right way.' To this he added: 'If you understand pure sciences you understand pure fact.'

While observing the 'tiny girls' lift and squat, he reminisced about the various certification courses he had once followed, and which he now declared were not worth his energy or money. One of them was an ACE certification,[111] which he completed in 1999 and for which there was no practical exam. It expired after two years: 'No exercise, nothing was required.' In Delhi, he signed up for a course with another fitness certification body that focused on strength conditioning. 'They say demonstration is important but it is simply multi-choice questions on screen. It is just a matter of saying right or wrong.' It was much the same story with GCC, a training institute that mainly provided online fitness courses. Even though the institute itself no longer explained what GCC[112] stood for, to Kaizzad it was Gora Chamri [White People] Certification. 'They are given tremendous importance in our ... It's all about Caucasian skin. Then I am free to say anything I want.'

Although not active on stage as a competing bodybuilder anymore, his powerfully muscular body featured prominently on the K11 banners that adorned the stage. He had taken the effort to prepare himself for this talk by employing some of his own workout routines and sticking to a strict diet. As a result, he was now able to show a tapestry of veins crisscrossing his upper arms, converging in one throbbing nodal point, which his rolled-up sleeves neatly emphasised. Meanwhile, the 'tiny girls' were employing his techniques and doing lifts and squats that seemed way beyond what they should be capable of, and the audience became increasingly more ecstatic. Sunny nudged me and whispered in my ear: 'That's what I was talking about.'

When I meet Kaizzad a few days after the Pune event, in his office in Santacruz East, Mumbai, I mention that I had been somewhat surprised by the aspiring young fitness trainers I met in the lobby. There were five or six young men and women in the process of signing up for one of the institute's courses. They did not look at all like archetypical fitness trainers. In fact, I joked: 'I think I look more fit than that.' Kaizzad said he was also not 'very happy with some of the backgrounds of the guys we see here'. He added, 'They are unambitious, stagnate, and they just do that one course.' A major problem, he felt, was that fitness is still one of the easiest jobs to get into. 'If you take a course with us, you get a job, it's that simple.' He estimated that a trainer can easily make Rs 40,000 to 50,000 a month—that is, with personal training—but Rs 70,000 to 1 lakh should be possible as well. 'It is the easiest field to crack.' Yet, there is considerable disparity on the floor. 'Initiative is key and that is often lacking with these guys.' He says that it is not enough to only take the basic courses but additional ones as well: 'You have to invest in that.'

K11 offers a 100 per cent job guarantee but doesn't place that on their advertisements because it is 'against the law'. 'We have these contacts with other gyms; all gym brands, we are there across the board.' Initially, K11 was a gym too, but since Kaizzad realised the potential in offering certification courses, the brand has focused on this alone. 'Fifty per cent is our passing rate at the moment. Interest and motivation are key in this industry.'

Although initially all the courses were offered only in English, they have recently expanded and are offering some courses in other Indian languages as well. 'Many go through a drastic body change when they are taking the course themselves,' Kaizzad says. 'Part of the money, they will invest in their own bodies. But one has to factor genetics in.'

## GENETICS ALONE WON'T DO THE TRICK!

Most bodybuilders I met over the years agreed that 'genetics alone' did not do the trick, even if there were bodybuilders known for 'being lucky' this way. Their refusal to think of genetics as crucial to physical transformation and competitive success underlines the centrality of knowledge. Victor's ability to capitalise on this knowledge epitomised success after leaving a promising IT career. The private-training business he continues to run is entirely built on his own successful transformation, from a relatively skinny youth to a bodybuilder with some of the biggest arms in the industry. But his body alone would never be enough to convince potential clients. As he often reminded me, 'Many bodybuilders have no idea what they are doing, they just follow their trainer's advice.' It was something he was deeply cynical about. In his experience, this often resulted in bodybuilders depending for supply on their respective gurus, who could not be trusted with such important health-related matters, he felt. Like many other successful bodybuilders, Victor was far from opposed to the use of steroids and growth hormones. In fact, he considered them integral to the sport. The problem, according to him, was that it required 'real knowledge' to use and prescribe supplements—something Kaizzad also agreed with.

It would be a mistake to think that any one of these bodybuilders held the key to fool-proof success. Their knowledge was largely empirical, gained on the way to their own transformations. If it had worked for them, it would work for others, they argued. And this was what they dangled in their clients' faces, sometimes making lofty promises about losing weight and gaining muscle. Akash was particularly critical of this, because he had observed up close how colleagues had made promises that they couldn't possibly keep. He blamed the gym's system of remuneration, but also realised that clients were often all too keen to take 'shortcuts' too. 'They think, with a bit of juice, they will magically get muscles.' Building his own body had cost him, but he had also gained experience and insight into the inner workings of the fitness industry. Since Akash's own objective was purely to excel as a bodybuilder on the international stage, he couldn't quite relate to some of his clients who seemed to entertain all sorts of 'illusions' about careers in modelling and acting, which he knew were very unlikely to materialise. Building his own 'bodily capital', he knew well how illusive and deceptive its properties could be.

# CHAPTER 4

# SOCIETY ON STEROIDS

*'The only people who see the whole picture,' he murmured,
'are the ones who step out of the frame.'*

– Salman Rushdie,
*The Ground Beneath Her Feet*

It has been a little over a year since I met Kishore. I last saw him standing proud though exhausted on the back of the lorry on the final day of Ganesh Chaturthi. Now I see his grinning face and muscular body plastered all over a van parked in front of the place where he operates an outdoor gym. A banner with pictures of people exercising hangs above the gate to what is ordinarily a wedding ground. Since it is low season for weddings, Kishore rents the place from its Chembur owner. Membership is Rs 3,000 per month, or Rs 7,000 for three, according to another banner. He had been in operation for roughly eight months, and now employs four floor trainers and one head trainer, as well as 'a girl' who does the administration and gives occasional dietary advice, for which she has obtained an accreditation course with something called the American Institute for Sport

Science. Like the trainers Kishore employs, she was born and raised in Chembur. While their own personal histories are of a working-class or lower-middle-class upbringing, the open-air gym is flanked by newly built, expensive-looking high-rises with aircon units humming quietly in the background. Across the road from the entrance is a shopping mall with all the trappings of middle-class life: a Levi's retail store, Adidas and Nike outlets, as well as a KFC and food court selling various types of Indian food, from north Indian kebabs to south Indian thalis. Kishore seems to have arrived at a place he could only dream about when we first talked about his plans, seated on the rocks at Band Stand in Bandra.

I find Kishore with his clients and trainers doing a handstand followed by a number of push-ups—a routine he repeats a few more times. A young muscular trainer follows his example, but the male clients in attendance shake their heads in disbelief. Meanwhile, another trainer is doing push-ups with one hand behind his back, his posture ramrod-straight. He is a relative newcomer among the trainers, but Kishore thinks he has promise. The clients have now started doing push-ups, using an old rubber tire for support; a little further, two clients are bouncing heavy hammers off another such tire. Their grunts are interrupted by occasional giggles and comments in a mixture of Marathi and English, alternating between mockery and encouragement. It's a strenuous exercise which is also effective for letting go of work-related stress and other types of frustrations, according to Kishore. In that sense, the entire gym provides an 'alternative' to the day-to-day lives of his clients, mostly professionals who spend inordinate amounts of time stuck in Mumbai's sanity-defeating traffic. It's dusty, grimy and sweaty, and the tools Kishore has his trainers employ for workout routines are the exact opposite of the trappings of their regular lives: airconditioned offices, artificial lighting and social pressure. 'There's always somebody leaving, somebody's birthday, some festival to take care of', as someone once explained, referring to the never-ending stream of treats being handed out.

As much as I know the 'wedding ground' to be a temporary compromise compared to Kishore's long-held ambitions of starting a fully equipped, high-end gym, he has made this current concept work so that it actually seems to make sense to sweat it out in this place. Like the Chembur bravura and goonda-infused roughness he sold at a premium to clients at Malabar Hill, Bandra and other upmarket South Mumbai enclaves, he has cunningly translated 'working-class' conditions—once integral to the transformation of his own body—into something that appeals to his well-heeled clientele. His own clothes are very much at odds with the gym and his trainers (dressed in the latest sportswear): he sports fashionably torn jeans, brand-new red Ferrari shoes and a tight-fitting blue V-neck T-shirt.

When we later meet in a dingy pub on the first floor of a rather decrepit-looking building in a side-street away from the main action, I mention how I was surprised not to see him in training gear himself. 'I have to set the style, man!' He adds by way of explanation: 'I should come first, then my trainers and then my clients.' What he means is that it should not just be his muscular body that stands out, but also his sense of style, in fact his entire comportment, exuding confidence and leadership. Placing a hand on his chest, he says, 'It's something I need to keep up, it's my business that's at stake, you know.' This is also why he did not want to meet at the mall across the road but instead at a pub a little further from the gym, where he knows it is unlikely that he will run into clients or trainers. 'They can't see me drinking, man. That would be wrong.' He needs to maintain a healthy image. He does not care about the men in this bar, greeting several of them like old friends, commenting cheerfully on the Old Monk and Thums Up they are downing and the greasy chicken 65 that is served on tiffin plates. 'They are different, not important,' he says, nodding in the direction of a table with young men who have just asked for another round of beers. He has known them for most of his life but would not expect them to join his gym. 'They are not interested in that,' he explains. 'They have other interests,' he adds ambiguously.

The other men in the pub strike me as a typical crowd for a bar like this: local Chembur blokes in their twenties, probably fathers already, neatly kept moustaches and the occasional beard, most sporting bellies of variable sizes. An old TV set mounted on the wall in the corner shows vintage Bollywood songs with the sound turned off, though still managing to have some of the men transfixed. It shows actors from yesteryears whose chest hair lusciously sprouts from shiny-red silk shirts, unbuttoned almost halfway, wavy black hair perfectly coiffured, and a voluptuous heroine coyly hiding behind a tree, which will soon stand for so much more. Maratha-born, Bangalore brought-up 'Tamil' hero Rajinikanth is probably the only leading man left who can still pull off looking like this, even if this pub is filled with men with body types much closer to these older stars than today's popular actors such as Hrithik Roshan and Ranveer Singh. Kishore stands out here; some of the regulars remark on his physique or casually pinch his biceps which he languorously flexes, smiling but not particularly keen in engaging in conversation any more than strictly necessary.

Kishore's muscular body and his sense of style radiate confidence, but his exuberance and powerful body also act as a façade behind which he hides financial and other worries that he cannot share easily with anyone in Chembur. Over the years, he has gradually become franker, seeing me as a non-threatening person to confide in, a firang who occasionally sails through Mumbai. 'Right now, I am making some money, but it is not enough,' he offers pensively, taking a determined gulp from his beer. He had been insistent on having Kingfisher Strong because he rarely drinks. 'When I have a beer, I want it to hit me, you know.' He hopes it will take his mind off things. 'Rent of the place is fifty-K [Rs 50,000], salaries eighty, another twenty I spent on advertisement, you know the stickers on the van, the banners, stuff like that.' He needs another Rs 1 lakh for his family, he says. 'Last month we made about three lakh and this month it'll be four.' The gym has about 150 paying members. 'Now we are making a profit but before that it was a loss'—something he is still recovering from. As a personal trainer, he used to make around Rs 1 lakh per month and he seems to be making an equal sum with his own business too. But there are many hidden costs that make his take-home feel less than sufficient. 'I have to look good you know, it costs money.'

Besides that, there are other factors to consider. 'This place is not stable, you know, there is no continuity', meaning the wedding venue. 'Three times a month, some wedding happens, and I have to take the gym somewhere else.' The occasional rain also complicates matters. Apparently, the owner makes Rs 2.5 crore on weddings a year. 'That man, he is now only realising that there may be more money in gymming, but how to convince him? He has to take a risk!' Trying to draw the waiter's attention for another round of beers and to order some food,

Kishore adds: 'This is not a real gym', at least not what he envisions for the future. 'I need it to be more luxurious, better equipped, all that.' But he also realises that because of the simple set-up, his investments are relatively low. He operates with a limited range of weights, some yoga mats, heavy balls for bouncing exercises, a few rubber tyres and a couple of kettle-bells. What the gym offers is a variation on functional training, partly because of necessity, but also because Kishore feels it is the 'best way to become fit'. His clients all live in Chembur, though they may not think of themselves as 'being from Chembur'. The newly built high-rise apartments have lured a young professional crowd to the area attracted by the relatively 'easy' commute to the city's business districts. The comparatively easy exercises that the gym offers appeal to them. 'Girls can do this too, they don't have to worry about anything.' Earlier, I had seen them go for a jog or doing some casual stretching and light exercises. According to Kishore, most women come for weight-loss exercises. 'Waffles are all the rage now, so they have too many of them, they get fat.' But he would never put it this bluntly to them. His female clients are like sisters to him, to be treated with respect, he says. He also prides himself for making the gym a safe environment for them to workout, something he goes to great lengths to instruct his trainers in as well. 'Outside, they face a lot, so inside, they should be able to relax about that.'

Although he is taking care of his ageing parents, younger siblings, as well as two children (aged six and seven), regular doubts are raised about the financial risks he takes. 'I have taken a lot of advance money from my clients,' he says, 'so I have to make this a success. Otherwise, there will be hell to pay.' His wife and sister are responsible for making sure that he is able to keep up with his low-carb, high-protein diet, preparing his meals in the morning so that he can have them at specific intervals throughout the day. 'They don't understand what I am eating but I taught them how to make it.' He also feels it is important that his family understands the middle-class lifestyle he envisions for them. His children now wear branded clothes; he is particularly proud of his son wearing Tommy Hilfiger and Benetton. In that sense, the childhood he is now providing his children with could not be further removed from his own, wearing his father's old shirts, which were already second-hand when his father bought them, and attending Marathi-medium primary education, where, he says, he had not learned all that much. Now, his children are enrolled in an expensive English-medium school, ranked among the best in the area. While this new middle-class life has offered his family the kind of comfort and luxury that was unthinkable for the previous generation, maintaining the current quality of life and making sure that their trajectory of upward mobility continues is a considerable cause for concern.

## A SOCIETY ON STEROIDS

How do trainers and bodybuilders deal with the financial precarity and uncertainty that comes with living and strategising toward new middle-class lifestyles? And how do their well-built bodies relate to this predicament? On the one hand, there's the muscular body that supposedly encases an equally, if not even more powerful, masculine self. On the other hand, studies have a tendency to emphasise how these muscles reflect uncertainty and an ambivalent relationship with societal expectations and changing gender relations. How does this paradox 'work out' in practice? How does the muscular body relate to the masculine ('confident') self? In India, this issue is further amplified by the way the Indian male has gradually taken centre-stage in debates about what is wrong with the country in general. Rape cases, street harassment and gender discrimination point at Indian masculinity's deeply ambivalent relationship with societal and cultural change. While this chapter does not deny that these are indeed significant problems, the popularity of fitness and bodybuilding also provides an alternative—perhaps slightly more hopeful—reading. It suggests that the muscular body is not so much an outcome of masculinity run amok, a way to reaffirm patriarchal relationships, or even 'simply' a product of changing gender relations, but instead one that reflects and actively engages with the changing nature of Indian society itself. As observed in the previous chapter, to a certain degree, the bodies of trainers epitomise a relationship with knowledge. This knowledge of transformation is directly connected to urban change and the transformational capacity of new India. Yet, as sure as these men may be of their own capacity to transform and guide their clients through a treacherous landscape of overconsumption and sedentariness, their own world is characterised by flux and uncertainty. In the fields of fitness and bodybuilding, revolutionary diets come and go; recommended workout routines change all the time; and there always seems to be some new miracle supplement on the market that could aid in weight loss, muscle growth and repair. The scientific facts behind health and fitness claims are inherently debatable and ambiguous, even though trainers claim that they hold the keys to the 'right information'.

While trainers were frequently 'on steroids' themselves, they voiced concerns over a 'society out of control', experienced as 'too soon and too fast', which they perceived their clients to inhabit. They felt that it was their duty to slow down their clients and have them adopt more reasonable goals. As a twenty-seven-year-old Bihari trainer, working for a high-end gym in Gurgaon (now Gurugram), once put it: 'They forget we are always in this gym ourselves, they only have to come here in the morning. They have a whole life outside. Then they want this body,' thumbing his fingers on the six-pack that was visible through his white T-shirt. 'It does not work that way,' he said, flashing a bright-white smile.

Even if trainers envision themselves as life coaches, beyond only providing 'fitness training', their knowledge was almost always contradictory, something the contents of male-oriented lifestyle magazines reflected as well. Diets, workout routines and the use of various supplements—rarely was there any consensus on the best approach.

Equally, if not more troubling, was the question of food safety and the guarantee that health brands, including those claiming to be 'organic', make. Protein powders were frequently used as a case in point. It was next to impossible to trust that the label's promises matched the contents of the box. As BodyHolics's manager Manish once explained it: 'I have seen this myself: they import these expensive branded boxes of protein, take out half and supplement it with some other powder!' As a result it was not unheard of for clients and aspiring bodybuilders to complain of unexpected weight gain. His trainers and clients only used the protein powder that he sourced through a trusted wholesaler and resold himself, making a 'small' profit. A gym owner in North Delhi made perfectly clear what he thought of the market for supplements in India: 'You have seen all these stores selling organic produce now, right? How will I know if that is the case? It's the same with these supplements. In India you have no fucking way of knowing!' As much as trainers and bodybuilders appeared to disagree on the best diets or workout routines, ironically, there was a clear consensus that it was hard to know if the supplements on offer were genuine or counterfeit. While the muscular body may exude trust and confidence in the effectiveness of workout routines, dietary advice and 'supplements' on offer, this trust also stood in direct relationship with, even directly building on, the inherently untrustworthy nature of the world outside the gym.

## Food Safety, Adulteration and Dependence

Food safety and food adulteration continue to be considerable concerns in urban India. Anthropologist Harris Solomon's important studies of food, fat and related illnesses in Mumbai (2015; 2016) touch upon issues of plastic usage and the adulteration of milk. Discussing patterns of food adulteration in urban India, his research assistant once complained that 'Everything is wrapped in plastic now ... Everyone is getting cancer here ... The chemicals go into food ...'[113] Like plastic, milk can also not be trusted, as it is often perceived to be diluted with unsafe tap water.[114] What is interesting is not so much the factual quality of these claims, but the fact that they exist and impact the way people reflect on their food consumption. At BodyHolics, such concerns had led to a growing preference for organic food among its members and dedicated organic shops had sprung up across the GK area recently. While no definite figures are available, the India Brand Equity Foundation (IBEF) estimates that India's organic food market will have increased three times by 2020.[115] An article in the *Economic Times* estimated the market to be worth $0.36 billion in 2014, and projected to grow to $1.36 billion by 2020.[116] Estimates of the size of the market for health products, including the sale of protein powders, are harder to get. Companies such as *Euromonitor International* do offer access to a country report for India's sports nutrition market on their website. However, considering how fragmented and complex the market is in terms of the number of brands competing, it is doubtful the report is worth its asking price of $990.[117] The visible presence of organic food shops, and the availability of whey-protein powders and health supplements even at kirana shops[118] across India, indicate a rapidly expanding market. However, even if this ubiquitous availability of organic foods and health products evokes the image of a more health-conscious India, those in the health and fitness industry are critical of these products. They would generally make use of alternative sources to obtain 'real' protein powder, high-quality supplements, and even chicken meat and eggs that were not loaded with 'hormones and other shit' as a certain gym owner phrased it once.

When it came to anabolic steroids and growth hormones, users and providers were even more outspoken. 'Getting the genuine stuff is an issue,' a young bodybuilder from Delhi (Girish, see chapter six) said. 'But I trust my trainer.' He had been on anabolic steroids and growth hormones for over two years when I first met him, and had experienced no side effects, something he credited his trainer for. Trainers, often referred to as teachers or even gurus, clearly made significant money through dealing in protein powders, supplements and controlled substances. They were generally men who had been successful bodybuilders in their younger years and were now operating gyms and related fitness businesses. In their dealings with younger bodybuilders, they relied on their past form and current well-being (health-wise, financially and in terms of social capital), emitting an air of confidence that could counter any doubt their 'students' might have. These trainers often functioned as gatekeepers, with the keys to the 'right' or 'correct' information about the most effective workout routines as well as genuine dietary advice. They presented themselves as reliable, whereas all these 'others' were cheaters. As such, they offered trust and confidence in a fundamentally unstable and deceitful world, where nothing could be known for certain.

## THE MASCULINE SELF AND BODILY WORTH

The issue of trust extends beyond the world of trainers and bodybuilders trying to carve out middle-class positions for themselves. The upper-middle-class clients of a CrossFit box[119] in Delhi—whom we will meet later on in this chapter—spoke to me about how their idea of an inherently untrustworthy, changing world impacts the way they relate to their bodies and workout routines. Even if muscular bodies, practically speaking, matter very little in their day-to-day lives as highly educated professionals, these Crossfitters are determined to emphasise their usefulness otherwise.

As was mentioned earlier, the muscular male body is layered with all sorts of notions that go beyond its aesthetically pleasing dimensions, or sexual attractiveness. Magazines such as *Men's Health* also discuss it in relation to it exuding professionalism, control and cosmopolitanism. It is generally the end product of a long-term commitment to strenuous workout routines and dietary regimes, that need to be reflected on in this light as well. The bloodied, callused hands of CrossFit's clients present us with an interesting conundrum here. A CrossFit box avoids air-conditioning and emphasises the need to recreate 'real-life' conditions inside. That these conditions are far more working class than what the clients in question are used to in their day-to-day lives doesn't necessarily point at a desire to involve themselves in working-class 'labour', but instead imbues their muscular bodies with notions of survival and control that add to their persona as high-end professionals who are in tune with the world at large.

There is a balance of risk and control at work here, which also runs through the case of Raj, a Chennai-based IT professional and team leader, and an aspiring bodybuilder in his spare time. I first met Raj when interviewing senior bodybuilder Srivat, whose recently established gym is located on the outskirts of the city. Like the clients at CrossFit, who obediently follow the instructions of their trainer, Raj had fully trusted Srivat to provide him with coaching and guidance. However, he also struggled with the question of whether he should invest in growth hormones to take his body 'to the next level'. Once he asked over lunch, 'What would you do, Michael?' His quandary was whether the risk was worth the cost in terms of his finances, health and even social standing.

Up-and-coming Tamil bodybuilder Shanmugan, who is considered one of the greater talents of recent years, helps situate Raj's story within a broader context. When I first met him, Shanmugan had already participated once in MuscleMania, billed as a clean and natural bodybuilding competition that was rapidly gaining popularity. However, he had never been a 'natural' bodybuilder himself, something his size and vascularity immediately betrayed. One of MuscleMania's sponsors, a businessman who runs several protein and supplement shops in Chennai, helped me understand how the idea of a 'clean sport' with a wider appeal, beyond the bodybuilding community, is hampered by an industry marked by uncertainty and disinformation. While the personal trajectories of Shanmugan and colleagues are revealing for how 'unclean' so-called 'clean' competitions are, its very claim of being clean and pure is ridiculed by bodybuilders who are (relatively) open about their use of steroids and who claim that one stands no chance of competing otherwise.

While the muscular body may exude masculinity—equated with confidence, trust and success—the path of transformation is strewn with potential challenges to masculine self-worth. Financial uncertainty, the inability to provide for one's family— even having to depend on family support—exist and are aggravated by the constant flux of Indian's urban environment. Risk-taking behaviour is a natural response to precarious conditions—created by rapid economic growth, changing gender relations, the social and physical transformation of cities—and the potential rewards are as spectacular as the potential failures. The muscular body is a reflection of all these tensions and contradictions.

## BUYING, CONSUMING, INVESTING

In *Who Me, Poor? How India's Youth Are Living in Urban Poverty to Make It Big* (2017), Gayatri Jayaraman paints a striking (though problematic) picture of debt-ridden Indian youth living in cities. While her usage of the label 'poor' might be jarring, considering the harsh conditions of poverty that a large section of the Indian population still experiences on a daily basis, Jayaraman's investigation of urban poverty and precarity does indicate a shift in thinking about how this might be an issue for another, more privileged, aspiring section of society as well. In her analysis, the decision to deviate from more secure income-generating trajectories often leads to financial insecurity. Having conducted numerous interviews with young Indians employed in professions as diverse as acting, independent consulting and software engineering, she found their stories echoed similar concerns of precarity, the burden of credit card debt, and the challenges of urban life and lifestyles. What runs through these accounts is disillusionment with what 'new India' has to offer and what it has delivered on so far. There's a certain buyer's remorse that filters through the pages— not in terms of products bought as much as investment made in the idea of an urban middle-class lifestyle. Jayaraman makes use of findings that emerged from surveys conducted by PRICE (People Research on India's Consumer Economy). For 2017, it was reported that credit cards were seeing an unprecedented growth in India, touching 32 per cent in 2017, a figure linked to higher consumer confidence levels. However, this is in marked contrast with a finding from another PRICE study that zoomed in on what it referred to as 'a true middle India'.[120] While the survey confirmed that there was rising confidence among this group, '69 per cent said they met their basic needs with great difficulty'.[121] PRICE's 2016 'Household Survey on India's Citizen Environment & Consumer Economy' revealed that more than a quarter of Indian households incur debt. And 27 per cent of these households have at least one outstanding loan. On average, their debt is Rs 50,000 in metros, boom towns and niche cities. Furthermore, 12 per cent have informal loans.[122]

Jayaraman's study touches upon manifold reasons for young Indians incurring debts, from simply overdrawing on their credit cards, which are increasingly easy to obtain, to education loans, unexpected medical costs, investments in alternative career trajectories and so on. Her findings echo those of a particularly insightful study, *India Becoming: A Portrait of a Life in Modern India* (2012), in which Akash Kapur describes the life of long-term informant Hari, a young, highly educated professional from a small town in Tamil Nadu. 'Like so many young Indians,' Kapur writes, Hari 'had great faith in the future ... [and] felt he was living in the right country, at the right time, working in the right field ...'[123] Yet, instead of a simple success story, Kapur goes on to narrate how Hari overspends, incurs massive debts and frequently changes course in terms of his ambitions. Hari dreams big, but his dreams come at a price.[124]

Both Jayaraman's case studies and Kapur's detailed and sensitive treatment of Hari echo the tension that characterised the lives of my informants as well. They worked on a sense of style that costs money and required a disposable income in the hopes of future returns on the investment made. But the future is filled with the uncertainty of having taken these risks, and the outcomes are far from certain. When things go wrong, they do so very fast and with great personal consequences. As Kapur shows, Hari's debts mounted not just because of shopping sprees but also because of a theft and because Hari came to the assistance of a friend whose mother needed heart surgery. His friend was unable to repay the loan due to an accident of his own in which he lost a leg.[125] An economic downturn in the IT sector, meanwhile, made it more difficult to find suitable employment.[126]

In a related study titled *Indian Youth in a Transforming World: Attitudes and Perceptions* (2009), the authors note that 'Wearing fashionable clothes is important for a large segment of the youth.'

They argue that fashion choices often reflect an identity that is aspired to, rather than real.[127] A short contribution by Swati Ghosh dissects how beauty and self-esteem are increasingly linked in metropolitan India, specifically Kolkata. She finds that the firm and slender body has come to symbolise self-confidence and security.[128] Ray Titus paints a similar picture in *Yuva India: Consumption and Lifestyle Choices of a Young India* (2015). In one of the final chapters, he touches on suicide, as it relates to issues of physical self-esteem, shifting social and sexual relations, and the stress of professional careers. Titus notes that India now ranks 'as among the nations with the highest number of suicides, especially among the youth and women'.[129] A psychiatric counsellor informed him how 'emotionally fragile the young people she meets are'.[130] The inability to deal with newfound freedoms, changing circumstances that impact relationships, as well as loneliness and the lack of social support all seem to be factors here.[131] Titus concludes that 'The new social realities of greater individualism, independence, and self-reliance haven't fully sunk in.'[132]

The speed of change in India makes the gaps in middle-classness and access to economic, social and cultural capital starker. It also highlights the widening gap between different generations. Almost none of the trainers and bodybuilders interviewed were able to rely on the support of their parents, not only because their parents had considerable doubts about the risks involved in the alternative career or business trajectory chosen, but also because they simply had no knowledge to share on how to handle the uncertainty and precarity that came with it. As self-made as many informants were, they were also very much on their own. The trust they may have otherwise put in family and community relations was invested in fitness and bodybuilding networks, which are characterised by a high degree of dependence on, and faith in, the trustworthiness of senior figures. A Delhi-based bodybuilder once shared a picture of himself dressed only in posing trunks, kneeling down with hands folded in worship in front of his trainer, whom he calls his guru, and who confers a paternal blessing on his head. While the image pays homage to the relationship pehlwans have with their gurus, it also implies that this bodybuilder, a successful trainer himself, is part of a network with its own hierarchy. He is compelled to literally kneel down before his guru's superior knowledge. This is, of course, a completely acceptable (and ritualistic) way of paying respect to one's teacher in his cultural sphere, but the gesture underlines how masculine self-worth, no matter how muscular its subject, is tied up with the relative worth of others in his sphere.

## MIDDLE-CLASS MASCULINE WORTH

One of the most iconic moments in the hit movie *Rang De Basanti* (2006) is a scene in which actors Aamir Khan and Sharman Joshi are perched on the edge of a wall above a water tank at Nahargarh Fort. They arch their backs to make it more difficult to maintain balance while downing full bottles of Haywards 5000 Super Premium Beer, a beverage known for its heavy alcohol content. Aamir Khan perseveres, while Sharman Joshi plunges into the water while attempting to finish a second bottle. Although it's a fairly typical Bollywood scene of male camaraderie, according to an article in the *Indian Express*

(29 June 2017), it went on to top a list circulating on Indian campuses of fifty-two different dares. The article was authored by Rimjhim Jain, a social rights activist based in Pune, who had brought together a group of young men—known as 'unruly' on their respective campuses—to discuss risk-taking behaviour and notions of Indian masculinity. Jain argues that the risks such young men take are attempts 'to prove that they were different—better—than other men'.[133]

Even if men like Kishore, Victor or Akash (see previous chapter) do not engage in the kind of risk-taking behaviour illustrated above, their bodies—which are after all exposed to various types of health-related risk—are very much oriented toward proving a point in terms of their worth and superiority vis-à-vis other men. Idealised notions of masculinity and manliness tend to be produced by and among men. While this often appears to take the form of impressing women, closer analysis reveals that what matters more is masculine worth in the eyes of other men. This doesn't mean that the 'female gaze' has not become more important in India,[134] but that it is equally important to keep in mind that attracting this female gaze is an important feature of being a man who stands out among other men.

Sociologist Bryan Turner suggests that in our postmodern predicament, we all have become flaneurs, surveying and consuming bodies while passing time (as if eternally stuck in an airport departure lounge).[135] His argument takes in the visibility of bodies in public, as well as how the body has become a product to be consumed, perennially on display, to be acquired and possessed. The ubiquitous presence of muscular bodies in Indian public space (on billboards) and in popular media (Bollywood, Kollywood, etc.) is layered with more than simple sexual attractiveness, especially compared to the way female bodies are presented in similar spaces. For starters, men on the covers of male-oriented lifestyle magazines are, in fact, depicted in a sexually attractive way, but rarely are they framed in this way for the opposite sex alone. While the final chapter will turn to its homoerotic qualities and same-sex attraction, these images clearly reinforce a desire to stand out amongst other men. Not to have a lean, muscular body not only means risking one's health, but also losing out in the rat-race in terms of gaining professional recognition, pursuing new job opportunities and being considered for promotions. In short, not being able to fully claim for oneself all that new India has to offer.

## BLOODY, CALLUSED HANDS

Hanging out at a CrossFit box in Delhi one evening, I notice Anoop repeatedly performing clean-and-snatch pulls, rapidly lifting a weighted bar all the way above his head with arms stretched straight. A trainer keeps track of the time and counts the number of times he repeats this. 'Stretch! Don't forget to stretch at the end. I want to see your arms straight. Count one-two before lowering the bar down! Don't be in a hurry!' The others who have joined Anoop are all evidently determined to do the minimum number of repetitions required. Sweat drizzles down Anoop's face, and his light brown T-shirt is almost completely soaked through; the absence of air-conditioning in the box is noticeable, to say the least. Having lifted the bar above his head one last time, he ceremoniously drops it to the floor and high-fives another member who has finished the exercise at the same time. Grinning, he shows me his hands, which are completely raw and bloody, the skin having scraped off due to the repetitions. He makes me feel the calluses on the pads where his fingers meet his palms, deep yellow in colour and leathery to the touch. 'This is what CrossFit will do to you,' he informs me proudly. Anoop wipes his hands on his off-white shorts, leaving smudges of blood, then pulls out his cell phone to take a selfie with a friend. 'It's the life, man,' he adds. 'I am feeling it every day when I come here!'

Anoop, a Kashmiri Pandit, is originally from Jammu but grew up in Delhi. Now living in the upmarket neighbourhood of Vasant Vihar, he works in Gurgaon as a talent acquisition consultant. Basically, he is the first wall to clear, the first contact point for new recruits, particularly senior-managers. He mainly sources prospective candidates through LinkedIn and Facebook, then sits them down to discuss job opportunities. Having completed a degree in hotel management from Mumbai, Anoop was employed with Hilton for three years, where he started as a management trainee and was finally appointed full manager. He subsequently went on to set up his own café and worked for a consultancy company that specialised in questions of urban development. His father is a civil servant and general manager with a government agency, while his mother is head of an accounting department. His elder brother is married and works for an architectural firm. Obviously from a privileged background, he is a regular at CrossFit, where his callused, bloody hands and scraped knees do not stand out among the rest of its mainly upper-middle-class clientele.

Anoop's gym habit was initially triggered by a health scare at a previous job. During a medical check-up, he was informed that he had better start working out soon—something a chest pain one night further underlined. He smoked and drank too much and realised that he could not go on the way he had. Joining

CrossFit had generated positive results within two months, and he had never looked back. He had no specific goals: 'Just to get fit, that's all.'

He now makes his way to the box on an almost daily basis. Basically a bunker-like room of about five by five metres with a small mirror on one side, the box has only ceiling fans for cooling. Its manager, twenty-nine-year-old Rajiv, is originally from Udaipur but migrated to Delhi when he was five years old. Rajiv graduated from Jawaharlal Nehru University (JNU) and his interests were primarily in the social sciences. His own fitness career started in 2004 when he enrolled in a boxing class and then joined a friend's gym in Green Park, another upper-middle-class neighbourhood in the south of Delhi. A 'small and thin boy' when he was young, Rajiv's motivation for working out was mainly informed by the desire to 'get bigger'. After a detour into event management, he completed a fitness certification course, joined a hotel gym as a personal trainer, and finally became part of the founding team of an international gym chain seeking to get a foot in the door in India. From initially making little more than Rs 8,000 a month, he quickly managed to double and eventually triple this. In 2010, he went abroad to 'up' his CrossFit skills and to do an internship in the US before returning to India and starting his own gym. Currently, he employs three trainers full-time, though he himself is also still employed two days a week by a well-known sports brand, where he takes care of the PR, recruitment and special guests that fly in from abroad to help build the brand.

Karan and Parmesh, two clients, often hang out with Anoop. Under the guidance of Rajiv, the three exercise together, challenging each other to do more lifts, chin-ups and push-ups, or simply stand resting their sweaty backs against the gym walls to cool down for a minute. In between sessions, Karan tells me he is involved in the family business, selling various spice mixes, and that he completed his MBA at UCLA. Parmesh got a degree in commerce from Delhi University (DU), after which he was employed for over a decade in regular corporate jobs and briefly stationed in Australia. While Karan joined CrossFit four years earlier, Parmesh has been with the box for just two years. For Karan, a regular gym is quite boring: 'A [normal] gym is crowded and offers no feeling of community.' He comes to CrossFit every day and considers the other members his 'true friends'. They even celebrated Diwali together recently. 'CrossFit is not about coming and going. Like you do in a regular gym. Here it is not competitive, it's collegial instead. We are here to help each other, you know.'

More recently, Parmesh had even become a trainer himself. 'I got laid off a couple of months ago and didn't have anything to do,' he says. 'So, I became part of this bunch.' He now hopes that membership will increase and that he can attract more clients for personal training. His view is that 'fitness is the need of the life'; it is what creates a change in people's lives. Karan agrees with this assessment. He feels it is important to have friends in the city, but when he came back from the US, he found it hard to fit in with them. 'Crossfitters hang out with Crossfitters,' he says. 'There is something about going to hell and back together.' He sees it as a bonding experience. The cheerful 'see you tomorrows' that ricochet off the walls when most members leave at around eight in the evening punctuate this sense of camaraderie and mutual bonding. Parmesh takes a little longer to leave, because he wants to show his new laptop to one of the trainers. Meanwhile, Karan is pressing a tissue against a wound on his forehead—the result of bumping against a bar while exercising—waiting for the bleeding to stop. He assures me that it is not too bad and jovially adds: 'All part of the job, man!'

An almost violent disposition towards the body characterised the atmosphere at the CrossFit box that evening, something underlined by regular, enthusiastic exhortations to 'destroy the body' and 'face the battle head-on', and the desire to leave utterly 'demolished'. While the CrossFitters were mainly highly educated upper-middle-class men in senior managerial positions, in the gym they were actually 'at work' and, in a sense, even 'truly' accomplishing something, it seemed. However, it would be a mistake to think of Anoop's scraped and callused hands as adjacent to a fetishised working-class masculinity. Instead, he saw his scars as compensation for the stress he endured in his daytime job, spending long hours in traffic commuting to and from work, and dealing with managerial duties and high expectations. As a counterpoint to all this, the box delivered something akin to instant satisfaction. As Anoop put it: 'It's such a good feeling when you get the session over with and it's done.' And his hands were a clear physical reminder that he had accomplished something. He didn't mind showing off to colleagues either: 'They are always so amazed to see them like this.' In fact, some would even ask to feel his hands, something he took particular pride in. He saw the calluses as an extension of, and a more visible reminder of, the muscular strength he had acquired working out, something that had no direct use in his work otherwise, nor was particularly visible while he wore a suit all day.

## Disciplining and Punishing the Body

Within the context of the West, the 'extraordinary fetishisation of muscles and muscularity in young men' has often been related to the demise of traditional male jobs that require physical labour and muscular strength.[136] Over time, the muscular body has come to be divorced from its specific lower- or working-class connotations.[137] The male-bonding and camaraderie we see in the CrossFit box could perhaps be taken as a sign of a crisis of masculinity. Faced with changing gender roles and expectations, men seek to reclaim their masculine selves through working out. The gym is then held to function as a space of homosocial bonding; it's where men can be among men without the nagging interference of women.

Notions of hegemonic masculinity, as initially conceptualised by sociologist Raewyn Connell (1995), play a particularly influential role in such reasoning. Principally a concept of power that points at the subordination and marginalisation of other possibilities of masculinity[138]—less oriented at 'masculine' success, bravura and competitiveness—the concept also raises awareness of issues of complicity. Hegemonic masculinity relies on other men not to challenge its exalted position within masculine hierarchies. As sociologist Michael Kimmel (1994) argues, failure to comply with social norms of masculinity (e.g. to be strong, successful, capable, reliable, in control), impacts the way men are evaluated and judged. Research has argued that the health of poorer men can be attributed to this.[139] Even worse, it could lead to violence and abuse of women, other ('less masculine') men and sexual minorities.[140] Following gender theorist and philosopher Judith Butler's notion of gender performativity,[141] it has been argued that masculinity can best be seen as a performance on a pre-set stage with only a few directors to be followed.[142] Macho masculinity takes up a domineering position here,[143] from which a normativity emerges that should be understood in terms of it needing to be 'proficiently performed'. In other words: it is something that one needs to showcase, show evidence and remind others of. Noted manly virtues are good health, physical and mental strength, stoicism, fortitude, courage and so on. As David Buchbinder, professor of Masculinities Studies, argues, 'many of [these] are integral to the calculus of power by which a patriarchal system operates'.[144]

## Indian Men Out of/In Control

Indian masculinities are a particularly complex topic to tackle, not least because of the intensely negative associations they evoke in a patriarchy-oriented society that features appalling violence towards women and entrenched gender inequality. When I present research on fitness trainers and bodybuilders at seminars and conferences, the question that is frequently raised is how my work relates to cases of gruesome violence, such as the 2012 Delhi gang rape. It is a question at a remove from my research, which mainly indicates men's willingness to mete out violence upon their own bodies. Yet, questions from the audience often follow a rather similar reasoning: surely these men's drive to build muscular bodies is just another example of failure to deal with changing gender relations, stemming from a sense of insecurity?

This assumption contrasts strikingly with gender relationships within gyms, which are rarely ever male-only. The CrossFit box described earlier had about 40 per cent female members, who participated in similar workout routines. The friendships Anoop, Karan and Parmesh had made 'in the box' also included these female clients, who held similar positions as they did in corporate India. In fact, gyms in India often turned out to be spaces that were characterised by a rather easy mixing of the genders. Many even offered self-defence classes, thus directly acknowledging the harassment women face in public space. Fitness training certification courses also came with specific classes on cross-gender relations and how to deal with female clients for whom direct interaction with a male trainer might cause discomfort. Women who worked out at gyms such as BodyHolics generally considered them a breath of fresh air from stifling gender relations elsewhere in the city.

Sociologist Radhika Chopra (2004) urges us to look at the relations between genders, as well as relations within a particular gender, in order 'to understand the contours of male worlds and masculine subjectivities.'[145] In line with this, anthropologist Geert De Neve (2004) cautions against negative stereotypes and essentialised representations of Indian masculinities.[146] He argues that in order to understand Indian male masculinity, 'men have to be relocated in the particular "social" and "spatial" contexts of their everyday lives through which they embody, negotiate or contest masculinities of sorts.'[147] Rather than arguing that their gym-built muscular bodies suggest an ambivalent relationship with the other sex, let's look at what the notion of physical transformation signifies, beyond the immediate goal of an aesthetically pleasing, 'attractive' body. If we think of the internalised 'masculine' self as an anchor for men to find stability and confidence, the context of rapid urban change demands constant re-anchoring because of the way it questions pre-held assumptions about what it means to be a man. Working out may be a way to seek some control over this, especially since it revolves so much around notions of discipline and perseverance. However, it is simplistic to think of this as merely another way of reasserting male patriarchal hegemony.

Trainers not only work with female clients—even touching them occasionally to correct their posture or to help with stretching and muscle release—but pursuing a career in fitness also requires them to break with many of the traditional ideas they grew up with. Lean, muscular bodies, laden with notions of professionalism and cosmopolitanism in magazines such as *Men's Health* point at physical control—not as a reinforcement of older, patriarchal gender relations, but as a way to seek out a new masculine self that is in tune with and even embraces societal change.

## PERFORMING A NEW MASCULINE SELF

The performance of masculinity—of any gender identity—requires an audience, whether great or small. The body is an unavoidable, constant presence in society, consistently performing the gendered self and what it is held to stand for. In an influential study on doormen and bouncers, sociologist Lee F. Monaghan (2002) shows how working out and disciplining the body contributes not only to a larger presence physically, but also socially.[148] Like the professional boxers of French social anthropologist Loïc Wacquant's study (1995), doormen can be thought of as entrepreneurs in bodily capital who have found a way to utilise their body to generate income and elevate their 'social' worth.[149] Not unlike gym trainers, the relationship doormen have with their bodies is principally practical, in that the work they do has a functional need for their muscular bodies.[150]

As in the UK, where Monaghan's study was situated, gyms in India do act as suppliers of doormen to clubs and pubs. A complicating factor in this immediate association between trainers and this class of professionals is the notion of violence and its class-based associations, something trainers are well aware of. While engaging violently with the body was something trainers and bodybuilders would often treat as a given, the idea that this muscular body would enact actual violence was perceived as deeply problematic. For the boxer, the main function of his body is to facilitate punches and provide strength to them in accordance with nationally and internationally approved sporting regulations. In contrast, the doormen's body serves primarily as a tool of intimidation—ideally never having to utilise its impressive actual strength. Yet, in India, trainers need to steer clear of even a whiff of suggestion with violence if he hopes to avoid the all-too-easy association with lower-class goondas. This he must balance with a physical masculine ideal that speaks of strength, tempered with the narrative of control and a successful transformation. And this experience of transformation, while it does attract clients, is first and foremost about the self; it is about answering a desire emerging from within, to build, shape and challenge the body—to see what it is capable of, what one is capable of.

Why torment your body? Why risk its health? Why seek to transform it into something that is not necessarily a healthier version of itself? Sometimes working towards a version that is not even considered 'attractive' by conventional standards? I ask Raj these questions over lunch in his office canteen, a food court in the IT hub of Manapakkam, Chennai. He has just shown me his latest photographs, which confirm that he is in excellent shape. His overall muscular physique is incredibly well balanced, with the various muscle groups all starkly pronounced, even if he is not quite competition-ready yet. It is his ambition to compete in MuscleMania Chennai the coming year, but he feels that, in order to achieve his dream, he will need to make a significant investment in steroids as well as growth hormones. Already, Raj is spending considerably on his body: on average Rs 12,000 or more per month. Half of this money is spent on food alone, Rs 1,500-odd per week, but this does not include protein powder, supplements and the money he 'invests' in steroids. He is contemplating growth hormones, which will cost him manifold this amount, but is struggling with doubt. Why should he involve himself in something that is both expensive and dangerous to his health? Health risks run from an acne-ridden skin to long-term cardiovascular, hepatoxic (destroying liver cells) and psychiatric issues.[151] Currently the sole breadwinner, with a wife to support (an IT professional herself but unable to work at the moment) and a school-going daughter, he is barely able to meet expenses as is. Why do it, I ask him point-blank. Why does it matter?

Unlike Victor of the previous chapter, Raj has no interest in becoming a personal trainer. It is 2018, and his career as an IT professional is going well and provides him with a stable income. He makes around Rs 80,000 per month, though half of it disappears in paying off the mortgage for an apartment he bought near his office. Furthermore, he has a personal loan of Rs 6,000 per month and his daughter's tuition fees to consider. He estimates that Rs 65,000 is the minimum he spends per month, excluding any 'additional' investment in his body. More recently, his wife has started voicing concerns about his health and asks him questions similar to the ones I'm asking him now. Meanwhile, he has taken a loan from an aunt to finance his bodybuilding ambitions, even if he hasn't told her exactly what the money is for. It paid for only five months' worth of various substances at the time, but he believes it propelled him to the next level; this has confirmed for him the fact that, if he is going to take any of this seriously, he will have to invest even more.

I met Raj for the first time while interviewing Srivat, the bodybuilder and owner of a gym in an up-and-coming area of Chennai. A number of luxury apartment complexes have come up here in recent years, which is a clear indication that the area is increasingly considered an alternative for middle-class families who previously might have chosen something more central.[152] In between, however, are still many plots of vacant land, some even dotted with grazing cattle, a reminder of the area's recent agricultural past. The area epitomises the reality of a new India that is often monotonous, a rapidly expanding urbanscape that devours former farmland, carbon-copying itself over more and more terrain with shopping malls and flyovers, interspersed by small shoebox-shaped concrete workspaces for small pharmacies, repair and grocery shops. Srivat's gym, which he set up two years earlier, fits in neatly with this canvas of somewhat slapdash urban expansion. While the gym is independent, similar ones belonging to national and international chains, such as Talwalkar's, Gold's Gym or Fitness First, are located nearby. At night, their neon lights blend in with those of McDonald's, Pizza Hut and KFC, while by day they often seem to hide in the background.

Srivat is Raj's guru and trainer—the person he trusts to provide him with the necessary steroids and growth hormones.

He has assured Raj that he really has the potential to be competitive on stage. Yet financial worries, health concerns, as well as his role and responsibility as sole breadwinner for his family continue to nag at this young IT professional. 'I got into this addiction,' he says with a hesitant smile. 'When I walk around, I can see these guys looking at me, they talk to each other, that guy has great muscles, they say.' Giving it some more thought, he adds: 'Or that's what I think they say.' People in office admire him for his body. He feels he has become used to other men staring at him. It's like there is always an audience, and even though there is no applause, he can imagine it. However, he also realises that he has come to depend on the attention. It's an addiction that translates into 'exercise dependence'.[153] Even though he is able to reflect on this critically, he does ask me what I think he should improve 'even more'. Raj could well be a textbook example of what studies call reverse anorexia[154] and body or muscle dysmorphia.[155] Struggling to reflect rationally on what his body looks like as he reviews its ongoing transformation in the mirror, in essence, Raj is dealing with significant body image concerns.[156] The risk-taking behaviour this triggers among fitness enthusiasts and bodybuilders has been well noted in related research.[157]

## TO SHINE ON THE STAGE ONCE

'I just want to do it once you know, shine on stage,' Raj says, having given various risks and constraints some further thought. The imaginary applause that comes his way on the work floor and greets him on the streets is not enough. 'People keep telling me I have a great physique. They put thoughts in my head.' Through the window of the canteen where we are meeting, I notice a large billboard with faces of mainly young men staring seriously ahead, flanked by a larger-than-life image of actor Kamal Hassan. It was probably put up by a fan club to celebrate the actor's achievements or perhaps his birthday. Raj does not read Tamil either, so there is no point in asking him. One argument runs that these flex billboards can be seen as a way for subaltern men to counter their marginalisation, by literally making themselves visible in urban space. In the case of Chennai, anthropologist Roos Gerritsen's pathbreaking work on Tamil fan clubs shows that such billboards position one club against others, all intended for the attention of local politicians.[158] Raj is a highly educated IT professional for whom local politics like this matter very little. Yet his desire to shine on stage, even just once, runs parallel to the desires of fan-club members or political associations who seek attention by plastering their faces on enormous billboards. Amidst an incredibly crowded landscape of commuters, pavement sellers, beggars and others, Raj stands out. Even if he himself thinks that shining on the MuscleMania stage represents an important next step, on the street, in the company canteen, or simply waiting for the elevator, his massively muscular body is already on display, catching the attention of everyone around him.

MuscleMania promotes itself globally as a premier natural bodybuilding competition. In recent years, it has made inroads into the Indian market as well. One day, I met one of its key representatives in south India, Anand Kapoor, at his sports supplement store in Thoraipakkam. He immediately made sure to emphasise that this was only one of three stores he operated, and that he was about to open a fourth one in Pondicherry. With representation in over twenty gyms, he claimed to be the largest seller of protein supplements in south India. Anand was originally with Citibank, completed his MBA with a business school in Hyderabad, and was working in a sales position where he was 'easily making the targets' and not 'facing a challenge of any worth'. From a 'typical business family', Anand said his father wanted him to become an engineer, though the 'business-side' always attracted him more.

MuscleMania was one of the events he sponsored in order to further his business interests in sports equipment and supplements. While bodybuilding as a competitive sport was on the rise across India, Anand felt that eventually it would hit the decline it had elsewhere. The main reason for this, he felt, was bodybuilding's association with substance abuse, which deterred 'ordinary Indians' from getting involved. MuscleMania offered an alternative: a cleaner version of the sport, drug-free and with side competitions for those interested in modelling or simply showing off their accomplishments (think 'swimwear competition'). 'People don't want to look like they have been using,' he explained. 'When a techie comes into my store, he wants the nice chest and to pump up his biceps for three reasons. One is that he wants a break in the movie industry; two, to attract girls; and three, because he is simply very passionate about it.' MuscleMania was designed to provide a motivational platform for this.

Throughout our conversation, Anand was particularly keen to highlight that MuscleMania was all about being a 'clean' competition, as opposed to the many regionally and nationally held bodybuilding competitions that were (and are) most definitely not free of drugs. While talking to Anand, I was reminded—not unironically—of Raj's predicament, trying to make up his mind about investing in growth hormones in order to compete in MuscleMania.

Ongoing interactions with Shanmugan underscored the difficulty in enforcing a drug-free competition. Twenty-four at the time of our first interview, Shanmugan was widely considered one of the most promising newcomers on stage in south India. None of his success had come 'naturally', not least because of his 'humble' beginnings and the sacrifices his parents had made for him to excel in his sport. Yet his occasional 'drug' use—crucial to his transformation and subsequent ability to be competitive on the bodybuilding stage—cannot be divorced from the actual 'hard work' and dedication he had put in his training routine and maintaining a highly specific protein-rich diet. He himself attributed his success to the 'transformation' he had pushed his body to undergo irrespective of steroids and hormones, something he could rarely afford. His participation in MuscleMania therefore struck him as justified, considering that his physique was mainly the product of his own perseverance, irrespective of the minimal 'help' he felt he had received along the way. In firm disagreement with Anand, who had occasionally sponsored him (or at least provided him with a steady supply of protein powders), Shanmugan was adamant that none of this was, in fact, about attracting girls.

Over a coffee one morning at a shopping mall in 2015, Shanmugan expounds on his desire to become a legend in bodybuilding. 'I want to compete internationally, to be on the international stage, maybe even [Mr] Olympia one day.' His ambitions were not unreasonable. 'Blessed with amazing genetics,' as Victor once put it, it was generally believed by the bodybuilding community and his fans that Shanmugan definitely had it in him. Funding continues to be a challenge though, not least in terms of accessing the right steroids and growth hormones necessary to 'up' his body. His father, who was once a talented artist and drew logos and advertisements for companies, is now a taxi driver. He had lacked the computer literacy required once the industry shifted to digital illustration. With only a small additional income coming in from Shanmugan's sister, a trained beautician, it is up to him to procure whatever he needs for bodybuilding by providing personal training.

Asked what he wants to achieve with his bodybuilding, Shanmugan quietly states, 'I want to show India the good fitness.' Something that resonates with Anand Kapoor's sentiments as well. However, in order to prepare himself for his very first bodybuilding competition, he had invested in 'drugs'. Lack of funding did not make it possible to repeat this for the next competition, but he was still able to claim second place. 'Without medicine I reached this much result!' He thinks he has his genetics to thank for this. However, if he wants to compete internationally, for example in Mr Olympia, he knows he has no choice but to let go of any illusion that he can do this without the use of drugs. 'We can't even stand in the shade of these guys otherwise.' He has incredible admiration for what these men are willing to do for their sport: 'They are awesome! Risking their life for passion!' He even goes so far as to suggest that 'they are the best of us', given the kind of dedication they are willing to put into their bodies (including the use of drugs). He feels that 'they are not using drugs to impress anybody'. Shanmugan's main worry about 'using' is that, once you 'get off them', it is easy to 'lose confidence'. He has heard about the bouts of depression some of his colleagues have struggled with as a result. 'You can use steroids, but you should be alive to enjoy the results.'

Looking ahead, thinking of the future, is crucial, he feels. 'What about your family? Most guys never think about that. They just want to look good.'

## MALE ACTION FIGURES

Shanmugan's transformation over the years has been nothing short of stellar: biceps ballooning, pectoral muscles expanding, his legs a dense patchwork of throbbing veins which his hoof-like calves accentuated even more. It's hard to imagine that anyone could believe he was a drug-free contestant. He was certainly already too large to be a *Men's Health* cover model, which was very sensitive about such associations. Yet a Bangalore-based high-end trainer—a recurring contributor to the magazine— once assured me that it was doubtful that any of the cover models had not 'juiced' at some point. 'It is not really possible to achieve that kind of definition without the use of something.' He was convinced of this. 'It rarely comes natural.' It bothered him that not only was bodybuilding itself not turning drug- free, but even fitness in general—at heart a health-improving activity—was moving towards drugs for the sake of aesthetics (meaning: the much-coveted six-part abs, biceps and the likes). He saw the dangers in this—the untenable expectations of the body that substance abuse, extreme dieting and risky workout routines created. In his own contributions to various lifestyle magazines, this trainer and journalist made sure to emphasise the 'actual correct way' of doing certain exercises, preventing injury and building a 'fit and healthy' body. To him, the answer to moving away from an 'unhealthy' emphasis on the 'perfectly' lean, muscular body did not lie in discouraging men to pursue this ideal, but to change the engagement with the transformation process.

When I met Shanmugan again at the competition, in which Victor also competed, he had grown even more in size and made it to the overall category, where he took third place. His physique reminded me of a study I came across a few years ago on the evolution of top male action toys from GI Joe and Star Wars over the period of 1965–1998.[159] The study found that these modern figures were not only larger and more muscular than previous versions, but that they had become so large that some were now more muscular than humanly possible, even with the help of substances such as anabolic steroids. Developments in international bodybuilding suggest that we may not yet know the uttermost reaches that the body can grow to and be shaped into. Victor's twenty-inch arms, Shanmugan's desire to compete at Mr Olympia and Raj's ostensibly simple desire to shine on stage are all products of the narrative of unlimited potential. Their 'success' in transformation contributes to the idea that this is indeed also possible for other men.

The evening I met Kishore in the dive bar near his gym, he suggested that he was gradually starting to feel his age. 'It's less easy now, Michael,' he said with a tinge of regret. It had made him softer on his clients; made him understand them a little more, as he put it. Meanwhile, he knew that his plans for expansion, or at least for a higher-end gym, relied on him keeping his body in tip-top shape. Like Delhi's CrossFit box, Kishore's gym positioned itself as a counterpoint to a society on steroids, not only with respect to the actual use of steroids but also in terms of a society seemingly out of control. Kishore, like his CrossFit counterpart Rajiv, not only acts as a broker of bodily knowledge but also as one who understands the pitfalls and predicaments of this world. While clients, often unwittingly, seek guidance about how to navigate their professional and personal lives, this jars somewhat ironically with these trainers' own ambitions.

The idea that India is gripped by a crisis of masculinity, compelling its men to pursue ever more muscular bodies, even to the point of pain, does not resonate with the way trainers and bodybuilders themselves engage with their bodies and the various insecurities, uncertainties and issues of precarity they face as part of their lives. Instead of thinking of working out and building a muscular body as a way to show mastery and dominance in the face of rapid urban change, my research actually suggests that working out, and the goal of a muscular body, reflect an acceptance of the reality of a society on steroids instead.

# CHAPTER 5

# CITY OF VILLAGE(R)S

*One day, when he was
about ten or twelve,
he asked his mother
'What is my caste?
Some boys in the
school were asking,
I didn't know what
to say.' The mother,
got up in the middle
of her supper, 'Beta,
if you don't know it by
now, it must be upper.'*

– Akhil Katyal[160]

It's around one o'clock at night and I am sitting on the back of Shivam's Bullet cruising through a nearly deserted Delhi. We are on our way back from a bodybuilding competition near Aya Nagar, in a village situated on the border with the state of Haryana. Shivam is in a jubilant mood, bordering on ecstatic, exuberantly singing various Bollywood songs about having triumphed in the face of obstacles. I am reminded of the final notes of the opera *Turandot* and its main character Calaf's final exultation when he is convinced he'll guess the princess's name by morning. '*Vincerò!*'—I'm going to win! Although Shivam has already had his moment of victory, sleep is just as far from his mind. Swirling across the road like a figure skater on ice to show me the agility of his motorcycle, Shivam laughs raucously, beating his chest with glee. He had taken the stage for the first time earlier today, and even bagged third place. At this moment, Shivam is invincible.

The competition started in the late afternoon and went on till well past midnight when the overall winner was crowned. Shivam had walked on stage, lathered in tanning lotion and wearing a tiny pair of posing trunks, accompanied by wild cheers from an audience of at least a few thousand people. The plot of land on which the competition was held had gradually filled up during the evening, and by the time the final category of a 100-plus kg was announced, crowd control was getting to be a challenge. The organising bodybuilding federation had to keep the increasingly enthusiastic and rowdy local youngsters at bay, so as to make sure the jury could still follow what was happening on stage. Taking third place had been beyond Shivam's wildest expectations, and leaning backwards, he checks with me again if I had also noticed the nods of approval he had received from the jury when the double biceps pose had been announced. 'Rajender-bhai was insisting on me participating,' he yells over his motorcycle's roaring engine. 'He said to me, Shivam, you should go for this one, I know you can do it!' He is superbly grateful that he took the advice. 'I wasn't sure you know, I had never done this before, but you saw me, na, you took the pictures?'

Earlier that day, seated in the front row as one of the audience's honorary guests and awaiting the first category of 55 kg to take the stage, I had noticed Shivam animatedly conversing with one of the organising federation's key members, Rajender Bainsla. Dressed in Adidas jogging pants and a tight-fitting blue T-shirt, affectionately tapping a motor helmet against Bainsla's chest to underscore his point, Shivam's silhouette reminded me of Captain America as he appeared in the 1940s and 1950s; six feet tall, an almost perfectly V-shaped upper-body, the kind of jawline that made it look as if he was capable of rescuing a damsel-in-distress, dangling from a building's ledge, at a moment's notice. With the competition about to begin, Rajender had to take the stage to make the first set of announcements, and the conversation was wrapped up quickly with a friendly slap on the shoulder.

Noticing a free seat next to me, Shivam sat down. 'Bainsla is trying to convince me to take the stage, but I am not sure if I am ready,' he explained. Considering his size, he had at least a few hours to reconsider. 'I am not sure, man, I have never done this before.' He was also apprehensive about the reaction from the audience. 'In these areas, people like this sort of thing,' he added vaguely. 'Now there are not so many, but they will be coming for the higher weight-classes, you wait and see.' Many chairs were indeed still empty. Behind the stage, the sky had turned a mesmerising orange and the air was thick with the smell of incense. As was customary with the competitions this particular federation organised, a richly decorated image of Hanuman had been hauled onstage and a pooja to seek his blessings was going on. Once completed, the master of ceremonies announced the first category of '55 kg bodybuilder'[161] competitors to take the stage. Cast in golden hues, twelve men walked on stage, their bodies a dense filigree of muscles. It wasn't altogether clear whether there was any volume to these muscles, or if the men were simply incredibly lean and wiry. Applause and the occasional cheer from the audience was followed by the jury's first instruction: 'Bodybuilder, first pose, double bicep, flex.'

## THE WORLD-CLASS CITY

Shivam had competed in the Open Mr Delhi Championship (2013), organised by a Delhi-based bodybuilding federation. The majority of its members belonged to the Gujjar community, which explained why this particular competition was held on Gujjar land. As rural as the setting may have felt, the place could still be reached fairly easily by walking down from Arjangarh metro station, via its exit on Mehrauli-Gurgaon Road. However, the lane leading up to the village was unpaved, at times just a condensed mess of dirt and rubble that had become a road simply by being walked upon. The half hour-walk from the metro station illustrated how quickly urban conditions can change in the capital. Multi-lane highways and metro stations serviced by trains connect the heart of the city to its outermost suburbs and satellite villages. The not-particularly-charming small lanes that I wandered through to get to the site of the competition were lined with half-built houses and workplaces, its inhabitants busy with repair and recycling work of some sort. It had rained the previous day, and although the sun had been scorching all day, there were still many muddy puddles. Tractors and other vehicles battled for space, women crossing the road had their faces covered in semi-purdah, and all around was the unrelenting cacophony that could provide a soundtrack for a village scene in a B-grade Hindi movie. It was striking how far away the city suddenly seemed, even though the metro station was only a few minutes' walk away.

It is difficult to coherently define Delhi. On the one hand, there is Delhi's centuries-long history, which speaks of no less than seven different cities over time.[162] On the other hand, there's the more recent development of satellite cities such as Gurgaon[163] and Noida—and the notion of the NCR, or National Capital Region,[164] that attempts to capture Delhi's ever-expanding urban agglomeration. The city's urban landscape is best characterised as an interplay of overlaying processes. The need to constantly redefine itself seems both integral to this as well as an inevitable consequence of rapid change. While the dream of becoming a 'world-class city' is frequently sold by policymakers, property developers and the media,[165] fuelling large-scale plans of urban intervention and change, the implementation of this dream raises serious questions about urban belonging and who has rights in and to the city. While urban planning has sought to deal with a ballooning population and inevitable urban expansion, sometimes 'urban planning' can also be held accountable for the chaos that characterises the reality of Delhi at present, as scholar and activist Gautam Bhan (2016) has argued.[166] Focusing on the forced evictions of the urban poor from their so-called bastis, Bhan situates this development within the broader context of a 'rapidly changing economic landscape with altered patterns and possibilities of employment, consumption, production and work'.[167] The trajectories of those inhabiting the city are uneven. The desire to become world-class caters to middle-class aspirations that mean little to the urban poor, and increasingly leave them in highly disenfranchised situations.

At the same time, the NCR's expansion is increasingly equated with what has come to be known as village-engulfing, the process whereby the metropolis integrates rural settlements into the folds of its cityscape, turning these former rural enclaves into 'urban villages'. In contrast with the urban poor of Bhan's study, a considerable number of villagers in Delhi's peripheral rural areas have benefitted significantly from the increase in the value of their ancestral land, especially the land-owning Gujjar, Jat and Yadav communities.[168] There's no denying the ubiquitous presence of brand-new SUVs cruising down dusty village roads in 'rural' parts of the NCR, local youth in designer jeans and branded shirts behind the steering wheel, bhangra blasting from the speakers. For the upper-middle-class members of BodyHolics in South Delhi, this was decidedly 'new middle class' behaviour. Even if they drove the same SUVs, wore the same sportswear, similarly obsessed about the latest iPhone or Samsung Galaxy model, and probably enjoyed Honey Singh's lurid lyrics, for the older elite, these supposed arrivistes were to be met with reservation and distrust. Interacting with Gujjar and Jat youth who were involved in bodybuilding or fitness, or simply hanging out with members of earlier mentioned federation, revealed a difficult, even acrimonious relationship between these communities and the upper middle classes. This was further underscored by the way popular media engaged with their presence in the city, often associating them with disruptive, dangerous or downright violent behaviour within the NCR. Caste was an intrinsic part of these discussions, whether it centred around demands for increased quotas in government positions or education, or land-owning disputes with violent outcomes. The debates that took place on TV and in newspapers were also to be heard, sometimes in coded ways, on the gym floor.

# Delhi as a City of Village(r)s

'Delhi is, after all, a city of villages,' Tejas, a regular member of BodyHolics, once remarked as we were talking about the city's many problems—from air-pollution to unsafe conditions for women. Tejas was involved in a family business that also included his father and several of his brothers, and which currently focused on various construction projects in Greater Noida. While the conversation had initially been about increasingly worse traffic conditions and the need for more flyovers—something always tinged with a hint of regret the damage to the city's aesthetic appeal that this entailed—Tejas was also seeking to explain the city's inherent village-like structure to a foreigner like me. To the suggestion of another client that it might be more appropriate to call Delhi a 'city of villagers', Tejas readily agreed, saying: 'That's what I mean, they are all villagers, after all.'

Noticing how the remark had left me somewhat uncomfortable, I was assured that it was all about attitude and behaviour. 'I don't mean these guys,' he assured me, nodding in the direction of Amit who was busy assisting a client with the leg-press. To Tejas and other clients on the floor, it was well known that Manish, Amit and several other trainers hailed from Chirag Dilli, an urban village with a strong Jat presence that had been part of South Delhi's urban landscape for decades already. While these upper-middle-class clients may trust these 'urban villagers', Chirag Dilli itself was an area they would decidedly avoid. Since urban villages are exempt from building by-laws and government permission to undertake construction on existing buildings, the chaotic nature of their set-up may be enough to deter the upper-middle-class gym's clients to venture out there. They also simply consist of entirely different worlds, cheek-byjowl as they are with high-end shopping malls and colonies. Like Chirag Dilli, the more outlying urban villages that had recently become part of Delhi's ever-expanding urban landscape were treated with suspicion because of how they contrasted fundamentally with the idea of the city's own upward mobility, challenging the very possibility of it ever becoming a world-class one.

What is it about Delhi's new middle-class 'villagers' that makes them a scapegoat for the city's many ailments? Why do they appear to stand between the city and its world-class future? The Open Mr Delhi competition provides a glimpse into the processes that bring the rural and urban into dialogue in Delhi. Those in prominent positions in the village were regularly called to the stage to be garlanded and honoured with various awards that reinforced their prestige and position within the community. Elderly men dressed in white dhoti–kurtas and turbans shuffled to the front, some leaning gingerly on walking sticks, others being helped by a younger member of the family. An all-male affair—even later in the evening, when the crowd had easily crossed a few thousand, there was not a single female face in the audience—the setting and context was decidedly rural.

In Delhi, the gap between what comprises the urban and the rural is deceptive, even when it seems as if 'villagers' can be confidently identified. The physical body also plays a role in how notions of the rural and the urban are formulated. While the muscular body may be integral to trajectories of upward mobility for lower-middle-class men, it needs to compete with older assumptions of who the natural bearers of 'such' strong bodies are. Within the context of Delhi, this association clearly befalls Gujjar and Jat men, belonging to rural/pastoral castes whose ancestral villages are located in Haryana and Uttar Pradesh. Considering the popularity of pehlwani wrestling among these communities, this is not surprising. In fact, Lord Krishna, one of Hinduism's most revered deities and a wrestling champion himself, is said to have been born into the Yadav community, still considered the traditional custodians of Indian wrestling. Casual conversations with BodyHolics's clients would also often bring up the milk-and-ghee-rich 'rural' diets of these communities, which were assumed to lead unavoidably to a powerful build. I was assured that 'such men' were naturally strong. A recurring question the moment people learned of my research was that surely most bodybuilders I had met in Delhi must be Gujjar or Jat? I had attended numerous competitions and events, and they did not confirm this assumption, but there was always a story gym clients shared of how somebody's trainer was a Jat-boy or how so-and-so was training under a bodybuilder who hailed from 'some Gujjar village'. 'These men' were not just highly visible in the city but also ultimately 'knowable'. While references to Gujjars and Jats were generally negative, direct experiences with individuals from these communities tended to be more positive. As a friend once told me about her trainer at the upmarket gym she was a member of:

> He's done incredibly well, that boy, he must be making what, forty-K per month? That's a lot for where he comes from. He drives down from his village [near Gurgaon] every day, you know? Takes him at least an hour or so. But he's never late and he's so polite. He always says 'ma'am today we will work very hard on your body'. But he's never pushy … not like some of these other guys. No lewd remarks, none of that what some of these guys have, that you don't feel secure around them.

## A City with a Village Background

The gym where the Open Mr Delhi pre-judgement took place was a towering multi-level structure with an enormous billboard featuring a bodybuilder, his fists held together, combat-ready, the veins on his arms as well as those lining the side of his head ready to pop. Inside, a small table had been put in a corner with two rows of white plastic chairs for the various jury members. The person in charge was an elderly gentleman with a commanding voice, speaking mainly in Hindi. Any bodybuilder entering the gym for pre-judgement would first pay his respects to this chairperson by lightly touching his feet and then bringing his hands to his chest. One by one they entered the gym in training suits, friends accompanying them, and stripped to their underwear, followed by stepping onto a centrally placed weighing scale. Little emotion was shown and even less acknowledgement made of the place they were in; it was clearly something to get over with as the actual competition would still be hours away for most. Since almost all participants would have kept an extremely strict diet for days already, eating almost no carbohydrates and sticking exclusively to protein-rich foods, while gradually reducing their liquid intake and even resorting to diuretics to make their muscular physiques look even more 'dry', it was no surprise that there was little energy left to spare for pleasantries.

Meanwhile, I had struck up a conversation with thirty-four-year-old Vikram, a regular trainer at the gym, though not an aspiring bodybuilder himself. Strikingly lean and broad-shouldered, he was dressed in jeans, limited-edition Adidas sports shoes, and a Lacoste polo-shirt. Though he commanded big-city style, while explaining some context for this particular competition, he seemed keen to highlight his own 'village background' as well. Originally from Khurja, a town around 100 kms from Delhi and mainly famous for pottery, his family had moved to the city in 2006. He was initially enrolled in a bachelor's degree in engineering, but later switched to mass communications and was then doing an MBA through distance learning. He had managed to improve his English after coming to Delhi by enrolling in a one-and-a-half-month intensive course, though mostly, he said, he had simply picked up the language by binge-watching Hollywood movies. These movies not only brought him the necessary entertainment and distraction from family affairs but also managed to teach him 'many things about the world'. Throughout, he emphasised how proud he was of his father, who used to be employed by the Uttar Pradesh State Road Transport Corporation in a supervisory-type of position, which he described as 'not so big of a job' but that 'still managed to get us educated'. However, he stressed that 'for a better living, you have to move out'. At the same time, he was not convinced that Delhi offered better living standards compared to his native Khurja. Village life came with a certain peace of mind, whereas the city offered mainly material comfort. 'My father didn't want us to work in the fields. He kept us away from that.' Now, making a living as a personal trainer, he hoped to start his own business someday.

Vikram was a spectator during the pre-judgement and the competition that followed. He was there just to observe, perhaps assist, but most of all learn how others presented themselves on stage. He knew their bodies would be judged in terms of certain key criteria such as symmetry, dryness (vascularity) and muscularity; however, he was also keen to better understand the 'total package' the jury was looking for. While discussing criteria that might make a particular bodybuilder a winner, Vikram pointed to a podgy trainer with rather uneven teeth who was sitting behind the reception desk, commanding a particular air of confidence. Apparently known as 'a Mr Gurgaon', he had put on considerable weight and was now a shadow of his former self. Vikram remarked that he had 'lost the physique' but that he was still a very respected figure in the bodybuilding community. He had seen pictures of what he looked like when he was 'at his height', pictures I had also come across online and which were widely shared and respected.

Most bodybuilders in the competition were from nearby villages. 'They struggle quite a bit to keep up with their diets and maintain their bodies as sponsorships are rare,' Vikram told me. The investments required were hard to meet for most, 'but also their diets are not always what it needs to be'. A Gujjar himself, he knew all too well how ingrained 'local' ideas of health were. 'Drinking a few litres of milk is not uncommon among these guys, you know? They're farm boys, they have easy access, they like their ghee and all that.' He himself knew better and stuck to what his trainer suggested, thus limiting his food intake mainly to vegetables, occasionally chicken (something that did not come naturally to him, having grown up in a vegetarian household), and his protein powders and supplements. 'It can be expensive, though,' he added with some regret but also a sense of pride. 'Now I can afford it.'

Stepping outside to see how the preparations were underway on the plot of land where earlier they were still busy erecting the stage, I met Manosh, one of the federation's central figures.

Dressed in the federation's suit-and-tie, he had successfully competed in events such as Mr Delhi and Mr Haryana over the years, but now considered his competitive days to be over. Employed as a hospitality manager with an international hotel chain, he combined his many responsibilities (from coordinating the airport-based sales team to overseeing the leisure operations, such as gym and swimming pool) with promoting 'the sport'. Originally from Haryana, he traced his roots to a village near Bahadurgarh but stayed in 'a village called Najafgarh', a Gujjar stronghold. Manosh said he simply considers himself a Hindu with no interest in caste politics. It is also not something that is supposed to matter on stage: 'Only the body counts when you are there.' As other members of the federation assured me, all castes and religions were welcome, something the names of those competing tended to reflect. But Manosh agreed with Vikram that 'many of the boys will be from around here', and those of Gujjar and Jat backgrounds appeared dominant. Some work out at the gym that was hosting this competition, 'others may go somewhere in the city'.

As for the local akharas, he was less certain about them. 'That is getting less now, they are no longer so interested in that.' In fact, he had heard that quite a few were now in the process of being converted to gyms or bringing in gym equipment.[169] 'Young guys no longer want to stick to that ...' which I interpreted as a thinly veiled reference to the akharas' brahmacharya ideal which promotes abstinence, not just of meat and alcohol but also of sexual intercourse. The influence of Bollywood was undeniable here. 'They all want the six-pack, eight-pack, so they go for that. A different workout is required for that, different food as well.'

Manosh used to train under a bodybuilder who was then preparing for Mr World and would not be present today.

He considers this 'three-time all-over India champion' his guru or teacher. This bodybuilder himself was coached by Bhupender Dhawan, another well-known figure in the world of bodybuilding. A Dronacharya awardee[170] for his dedication to bodybuilding, Bhupender was, in fact, never a bodybuilder himself. His Dronacharya gym chain remains a well-known source for bodybuilding talent in the city, and it is where Manosh used to work out. He fondly recalled his own posing days as we watched young bodybuilders enter and exit the gym, often looking listless if not downright sleepy. 'When they get on stage, you will see a whole different personality,' Manosh guaranteed me. 'Then they will give a good show.' He was sure of that. 'But now they won't show it because they haven't eaten anything. They will be reserving their energies to give a good stage presence.' The way they presented themselves on stage could make a huge difference, and for the jury, this often meant taking difficult decisions. 'Sometimes you have to give a bodybuilder less although their physique is quite good. On stage he has to be like an actor, they are a different person altogether.' But this did not just apply to what they did on stage, he felt. 'It's also when they want to make a living out of this, they have to understand how to present themselves to clients.' They will not all have successful careers, he felt. 'Some of these guys can't talk, they don't know English very well.' For information about their workouts 'these guys' would rely mainly on their trainers 'who can tell them anything', making a rather oblique reference to the copious use of steroid and growth hormones among bodybuilders. 'But if they are from the villages, they also sometimes don't know how to behave in the city, that is the problem,' he said. With a father who had always made sure that his son got an 'English-medium' education, he felt he had never struggled with this himself.

Both Vikram and Manosh were born, brought up and continued to live in villages, but there isn't anything that makes them villagers per se, even if their village origins remain an integral part of the story they narrate about themselves. This is much less the case when it comes to their caste background, which only features peripherally in these stories. As much as their personal trajectories and family histories point to 'being Gujjar', the aspect of their lives that both men emphasised is the route from village to city that they 'traversed', subsequently making a living away from home and community and struggling to acquire the necessary education and knowledge 'to survive'. Now successful professionals, they reflected on the bodybuilding competition with a certain disdain, even if they were involved in the organisation themselves. Vikram expressed this in his opinion of the participants—'local boys from nearby villages'— of whom he did not have particularly high expectations. 'But there will be some good guys on stage, you'll see what I mean.' Manosh was less outspoken but seemed puzzled by the location of the competition. 'They might not like to come to a village from the city,' he thought. Moreover, holding the competition in an open field would require waiting for the sun to go down, considering it was still very hot during the day. 'It's better to do it inside, but these people wanted it to be done here. They take some pride in that. It gives their village a good standing.'

## CASTE AND LAND POLITICS

There is something categorically fallacious about the dichotomy of the rural and the urban.[171] In the case of Delhi, the urban and rural are decidedly connected and entangled. Sociologist Sanjay Srivastava (2015), of the Institute of Economic Growth in Delhi, speaks of 'entangled urbanism' when describing the complexities of urban development and planning as well as the many groups of stakeholders involved across the socioeconomic spectrum. In research that deals with the complexities that emerge from such entanglements in India, the focus is often on the urban poor and the way they negotiate everyday life in the city, struggling against forced displacement and evictions, demanding a home to live in and a dignified life, while faced with an often-venal state machinery's ambitions of world-classness.[172]

International development and global urbanisms scholar Ananya Roy (2011) uses the idea of subaltern urbanism to discuss the various strategies the urban poor engage in to protect their rights and livelihoods. As with Gautam Bhan's seminal work on the topic, the focus is on those who are in particularly vulnerable positions. While 'village engulfing' follows a different trajectory, in that it does directly (financially) benefit the landholders involved, it not only leaves a sizeable segment of the local population (often 'landless' Dalits) in a disenfranchised position, it also ushers in big-city dynamics and expectations that rural communities are often ill-prepared for.

While this chapter focuses on Gujjar and Jat land-owning communities and their rural-to-urban trajectories, parallels can be drawn with the Thevar and Gounder (Kongu Vellalar) castes of Tamil Nadu, the Lingayats in Karnataka and Maharashtra's Marathas. It is also not that much of a stretch to draw comparisons between Gurgaon and other post-1991 urban expansions and transformations, such as Bangalore's Whitefield or Calcutta's New Town.[173] Related regional ('rural') caste groups have all pushed for increased reservation quotas and/or a change in hierarchical designation (for instance by seeking Other Backward Caste status) at some point. Yet there are obvious differences as well, the most important being that, compared to Delhi, the urban expansion of cities such as Bangalore, Hyderabad or Mumbai has intruded much less on high-value agricultural land, and often involved engulfing areas that could already be characterised to a certain degree as 'urban'.[174]

It was the 1961 Delhi Master Plan that initially set the tone for the city's urban planning and policy.[175] Village engulfing needs to be understood as an inevitable outcome of what was set in motion then. The Delhi Development Authority (DDA), responsible for executing the plan, annexed agricultural land and absorbed villages in its wake, as a result of which an initial forty-seven villages in 1961 had increased to 135 in 2013.[176]

Gurgaon in Haryana is probably the most famous case of how spectacularly vast and fast the rural-to-urban transformation has been in the NCR. A small agricultural town till the mid-1980s and the least developed of all of Delhi's satellite towns, it would transform into an international hub with distinctly 'Americanising' ambitions post 1991.[177] It is currently one of India's major outsourcing hubs, housing a number of multinationals, ranging from Alcatel and IBM to British Airways, General Electric, General Motors and Nestlé.[178] Besides that, the 'city' has invested heavily in Special Economic Zones to appeal to international companies—all made possible by the buying up of land from peripheral villages.[179] While this has enriched land-owning communities, a complaint regularly heard is that grazing (gauchara) land has disappeared, leaving a younger generation without much purpose in life,[180] something that contributes to the impression of aimless youth with new wealth to spend but without the necessary sociocultural capital to fit in with an older (formerly wealthier) upper middle class.

A comparative case can be made here for Delhi's other sizeable satellite town, the planned city of Noida in Uttar Pradesh. The direct product of a law that came into being on 17 April 1976, the basic aim of Noida was to shift industry away from Delhi. However, Noida ended up growing much faster than expected, and in 1989 an initiative was undertaken to extend Noida into what is now called Greater Noida. While Noida was a carefully planned city, Greater Noida engulfed manifold villages, which were swallowed up by large-scale urban planning and building activities in rapid succession. As with Gurgaon, the increase in land value, the backdrop of caste politics, and the complex involvement of the state, large-scale real-estate developers and myriad other players have created a volatile situation that not rarely leads to violence and bloodshed. While on the face of it they ought to be natural allies, the Gujjar community and the hierarchically somewhat higher-placed Jat community[181] have rarely joined hands as landowners with joint interest, as sociologist and public intellectual Dipankar Gupta (2000) also notes. To the contrary, within the context of urban expansion and increased land value, both communities often appear to be competitors. The ensuing conflicts could be understood to at least peripherally contribute to the continued urban-middle-class perspective of these communities as boorish, feudal and socially backward.[182] A prominent role in the way perceptions are shaped is not just the way both communities regularly make headlines for their involvement in caste-related violence, but also for their involvement in large-scale agitations and disruptions. While this is a simplistic sketch of a highly complex situation, it aims only to be impressionistic, attempting to portray the perception or idea of Delhi as a city of villages, villagers and village interests. The point I seek to make should not be understood as to vilify said caste groups, who themselves are victims of state-sponsored and privately initiated developments, but to show how the perception of 'who they are' continues to colour relations and constrain upward mobility.

## THE FRAGILITY AND PRECARITY OF THE CITY ITSELF

Jat-led actions in particular are frequently held up as evidence of the fragility of and the ease with which the smooth functioning of Delhi can be disrupted. In 2016, Delhi faced a severe water crisis when Jat protesters forcibly closed the inlet gates to Munak Canal, one of the city's main water sources, carrying as much as 60 per cent of its water.[183] It has become increasingly common to employ the shorthand of 'Jat agitation' to refer to such actions and to question their justifiability by labelling it as 'quota blackmail' and claiming that the city is being held at ransom.[184] Often invoked is the argument that Jat and Gujjar communities are comparatively well-off, with reports citing ostentatious consumerism and lavish spending on spectacularly flamboyant weddings. Making note of guest lists running into the tens of thousands, *The Times of India* remarked on dowry gifts of cars and real estate, and that even choppers were not beyond the realm of possibility.[185] The framing is mainly one of unbridled ostentation run amok, lacking sophistication and restraint. Already in 2007, author and activist Primila Lewis described the Gujjar community as having been 'hurled into raging consumerism of liberalising, globalising India singularly ill-equipped to deal with it.'[186] This assertion followed a few weeks after Gujjars had laid siege to various entry points of

Delhi and blocked railway tracks in order to demand Scheduled Tribe status in the state of Rajasthan and 5 per cent reservation in government jobs.

In an insightful study, with a focus on western Uttar Pradesh, beyond Greater Noida, researcher Satendra Kumar (2011) concludes that there are no significant differences in terms of socio-economic status between Gujjar, Jat and Yadav communities. In terms of education, all three can be considered backward, with high levels of illiteracy and low college attendance.[187] While Jats are known for having accumulated considerable wealth by selling off farmland, Bhatia Singh notes that, with the continuous subdivision of landholdings due to prevailing inheritance practices (which means land has to be divided among all sons), average plot sizes have declined over time.[188] In effect, this means that while families as a whole may have profited from selling off land—with 'capital' having to be shared among many family members—'individual' spending power is a different matter. Another consequence of selling off farmland has been a diminished sense of masculine self-worth for young Jats.[189] While wealth may have increased as well as opportunities for consumption, there is 'simply' less to do at the same time. As sociologist Radhika Govinda (2013) describes it, in the context of Shahpur Jat, the urban village in South Delhi that was the location of her research: 'Young Jat men can be seen strutting around in Nike and Reebok T-shirts, tight enough to reveal their big biceps, mobile phones in hand, with loud techno and trance music blaring from their swanky cars.'[190] 'Eve-teasing' is a favourite pastime, but she also notes excessive drinking and visits to Delhi's red-light areas as causing the village ambience to deteriorate. Spending time at home with family is clearly no longer the norm, Govinda concludes.

Similarly, the Gujjar community more commonly makes headlines due to caste violence, especially as part of clashes with the (Dalit) Jatav community with whom they often share villages. Invariably, such accounts boil down to property disputes, for instance in Ramgarh village, which made headlines in 2012. Gujjar men had gone to the village's Dalit colony armed with sticks, country-made pistols and axes and beaten up men, women and children. The conflict at the heart was a local land-allocation issue involving panchayat land that had been allotted to sixty Jatav families for houses or cattle-sheds. Instead, the Gujjar gram pradhan, or panchayat head, decided to occupy the land himself. The razing of the colony was clearly meant to teach the Jatavs not to interfere in the grander scheme of things. With many Jats having sold their land and Gujjar families in the process of doing so, Jatav families have been left with little means to earn an income. Most continue to be landless, mainly seeking employment as farmhands. A *Frontline* article that presented a detailed analysis of the case reveals the broader context: 'Around Ramgarh, a private construction company has acquired most of the lands to build a mega city consisting of housing societies, shopping malls, private schools and hospitals and large sports facilities.'[191] According to the article, most Jat families had already sold their land to the company that was supposed to build the proposed town called Sushant Megapolis. Local Gujjar families were most likely going to follow suit.

The case of Ramgarh village reminded me of a similar one a few years earlier in Kanavani, which also involved a Gujjar–Jatav clash. Here, the property dispute involved an ex-pradhan and members of both communities.[192] It revolved around the ownership of sixty-five square metres of land which the former village head, a Gujjar, together with a brother and nephew, sought to claim ownership of by raising a token construction.[193] The Jatav community had objected to this after which it had come to an all-out confrontation. A twenty-two-year-old was shot dead and several homes and vehicles destroyed. The man who lost his life was a recently married 'B.Com student' and a Gujjar. As retaliation, a Dalit school was bulldozed to the ground the same night, and several families had to flee their homes for fear of further violence. Before the clashes, the family of the murdered Gujjar youth and the two main Jatavs involved in the dispute had been on good terms and had worked together for years in the real estate business.[194]

Ramgarh lies just beyond Greater Noida, while Kanavani is located within Noida's boundaries, not too far from Ghaziabad. Both are within the now established parameters of the NCR.

The agitations, conflicts and bloodshed sketched briefly here do not in the least do justice to the complexity of inter-caste relations, ownership disputes, or the politics that cause these divides to play out in these specific ways. All it attempts to do is briefly sketch the interplay of factors that complicate the deceptively simple rural–urban dichotomy. The urban is constantly present in these 'rural' issues, while rural complications leave their mark on the city as well. Besides, the way such agitations and bloodshed get reported on leaves its mark on how Gujjar and Jat men are regarded (often with suspicion) more generally. The biographies and day-to-day experiences of lower-middle-class men in Delhi reflect this quandary, in that trajectories of upward mobility often require negotiating and renegotiating the relationship between rural and urban, especially in terms of ideas of masculinity. This is not so much about actually moving out of one's ancestral village or the experience of the village becoming part of the city, but rather about the realisation of what 'the city' and 'urban life' itself are held to stand for.

On the one hand, bodybuilding, with its highly specific associations with massively muscular bodies, resonates a village ideal—that of the pehlwan or well-built rural figure, a product of the land and diets rich in ghee and milk—on the other hand, this bodybuilder's body also has the potential to appeal to an urban upper-middle-class clientele with its promise of transformation. The body thus reflects the potential of the city as well as its limitations.

## BODYBUILDING FROM VILLAGE TO CITY

A few weeks after his win, Shivam takes me to Rajender Bainsla's house in a busy market area of South Delhi, not too far from Kalkaji mandir. He was still riding high on claiming third place and had shown the pictures to all his friends and colleagues. During the day, Bainsla runs a women's-only gym but is also involved in various other fitness-related business ventures as well. Shy about his English, he is mostly quiet, only occasionally interjecting as Shivam holds forth on Delhi's bodybuilding scene. Seated on red plastic chairs in a spartanly decorated room with a lone poster of Lord Hanuman on the wall, he is keen to make me understand the mammoth contribution Bainsla has made to the sport and to him personally. 'No bloody coach knows all this medical stuff like he does,' he says, referring to protein intake, supplements and steroids use. 'I will explain each and every one thing to you,' he adds confidently.

'There is this tag that we are all poor people here. Why is that?' I interpret this to be an echo of the impression Shivam himself has of Delhi's bodybuilding scene. Born in a Brahmin family and brought up in Inderpuri, a somewhat affluent suburb in Delhi, he belongs to the 'middle' of the middle classes, and is employed with an agency tasked with investigating corruption-related issues. He has had an English-medium education, and his fluency impresses and even intimidates Bainsla, who usually has an impressive effect on others himself. Vipin, a younger cousin of Bainsla's, who has just joined us, and is one of his disciples, also treats Shivam with reverence. Eager to continue his laudation of Bainsla's many accomplishments, Shivam says: 'Bainsla-ji here, he has been here and he has done nothing but raise the name of bodybuilding!' Vipin agrees, nodding ardently. 'It is his goal to produce bodybuilders like Shivkumar,' he says, referring to a well-known senior bodybuilder who often makes special appearances at local bodybuilding competitions. 'He has trained more than hundred bodybuilders!'

For Shivam, Shivkumar is an idol whose form he can only hope to approach one day. But it is not just his physique that Shivam admires: 'You know, in 1994 he was only a slum-guy?' Bainsla smiles in agreement. 'He did not get a single meal per day. He did not even have two, three rupees to spend per day!' Turning to Bainsla, he says something in Hindi which translates as 'if nobody is there for you, God is there'. 'But God will not come by himself, God will always come as a person.' And that's how Bainsla's entry into Shivkumar's life should be interpreted, according to Shivam. 'He saw some spark in that guy and he decided to make him a personal champion. He decided that on the spot.' Apparently, Shivkumar was not involved in bodybuilding at all before this. 'I have no words for his dedication that way. He had given him money, shelter. He has done that for so many. Shivkumar was normal at the time, not a single muscle!'

Throughout Shivam's oration, Vipin is vigorously shaking a plastic flask filled with water and protein powder, the smell of vanilla wafting every time he unscrews the lid to take a sip. He wears a white vest, black shorts and faded red flip-flops, and the harsh tube light that illuminates the room ricochets off his bald head. A neatly kept moustache with the edges pointing upward complements a carefully cultivated image that combines the rural strongman with the B-grade Hindi film actor ready to rid his village of corrupt police officers and an evil property developer. Even though his body lacks the kind of definition required to be competitive, his look makes him a popular presence at bodybuilding competitions. An ostentatious presence at such competitions, he is usually dressed in jeans, cowboy boots and a white shirt, the sleeves neatly rolled up to reveal his powerful biceps, a golden bracelet on one wrist and an expensive-looking watch on the other. Vipin keeps the top three or four buttons of his shirt open to give his sprouting chest-hair space to breathe. On occasion, he even carries a small silver gun, deftly holstered and clipped to his belt, much to the awe and admiration of those in the audience. I know it bothers Shivam who finds it 'too village-like', but there is a palpable effect on the audience each time he makes an appearance. He is clearly flaunting an image that appeals as much as it causes confusion. Is he perhaps really an underworld figure? Might he be aspiring for a role in the movies? What precisely is he trying to say? I had heard members of the audience gossip about this but was never quite sure myself, and Shivam admitted once that he wasn't either. For all his presence, Vipin was never much of a talker. Instead, it is Shivam who talks about his financial troubles.

'You know that his family lives thirty kilometres from this place?' Shivam gently pats Vipin's back. 'But he rents a place here in this building because one day he will be a big champion.' Apparently, he has a wife and two children back in the village, which is located somewhere in Greater Noida. 'It's very different there, you should see it.' Shivam shakes his head as if in disbelief. 'One day we will go there, we will all go together and make a trip out of it.' Vipin seems to like this suggestion. While Bainsla has left the room to take care of some business, Vipin is encouraged to take off his singlet and flex his muscles to showcase the progress he has made. 'Wow, what a physique,' Shivam says in admiration. 'The only thing he needs to do is shave his body. He is too hairy.' Vipin flexes a few more times, which leads Shivam to conclude that 'he will be such a big star, this guy'.

As always, the conversation turns to the lack of recognition of bodybuilding as a serious sport by the Indian government. Shivam says, 'It's such a craze to be in this game. But the government is not taking care of us at all.' In fact, he is contemplating approaching the media about this. 'I am gonna make them hear about this!' Pointing to Vipin, he continues: 'Look at the investment he has made in his body. He has such a big body now!' He takes Vipin's phone and starts browsing through his pictures to show the progress he has made. Various pictures scroll past, all invariably with Vipin posing on the hood of a Jeep or next to an SUV, the sprawling UP-countryside behind him. In one, he is standing next to a cousin who has a bulky physique; Vipin informs me he is a well-known pehlwan. In another, the famous Shivkumar is flexing his muscles at the airport, on his way to a competition in Mongolia or perhaps another destination, Vipin is not sure.

Vipin and Shivam have clearly known each other for a while, but are obviously from very different backgrounds. Shivam's English is fluent, Vipin is barely able to string a coherent sentence together in the language. Shivam is from the city, while Vipin's village background is constantly emphasised, even though he resides in South Delhi. In a mixture of English and Hindi, haltingly Vipin explains: 'I am so messed up with life. This is a bad test.' He is finding it hard to put into words what he is going through. 'My family, they are expecting much from me.' Shivam takes over and explains that, now that Vipin is married, he is supposed to put the well-being of his parents front and centre, but his bodybuilding aspirations are in the way. 'In our culture, we all appreciate that, after marriage, he has a bride and gives comfort to his father and mother.' However, the predicament is that Vipin is 'totally focused on becoming big'. That way, he will be able to 'show true respect to his parents'. His wife takes care of his parents, while Vipin focuses on his bodybuilding career, which he combines with providing fitness training. 'He's always concerned not to neglect them as a man'—of that Shivam is certain.

As landlords, the family has made 'some big investments', as Shivam puts it. They are involved in construction projects in Greater Noida, but have also sold off considerable plots of land. There is money, Vipin seems to suggest, but not necessarily purpose. 'He is giving it his all,' Shivam explains, 'but it is not easy, being a bodybuilder, wife and kids at home, back in the village.' This is something Vipin definitely agrees with, but he also seems befuddled with how Shivam heaps praise upon praise. Throughout our conversation, it is hard not to notice how Shivam takes the upper-hand, emphasising Vipin and Bainsla's trajectory, their limited English language skills and humble village-like upbringing, while underlining their successes. Bainsla's assertion that it is his aim 'to improve the bodybuilding and bodybuilders in India' is quickly followed by Shivam's avowal and clarification that it's Bainsla's intention 'to take it to the height of success'. And Shivam is keen to be part of this himself, knowing they can use his skills and contacts. 'I am gonna change the way. I am gonna make them see about the game,' meaning the government as well as the public at large.

Bainsla and his direct associates' involvement in the local bodybuilding federation and related fitness business ventures remained relatively constant over the years I knew them, profiting from the sport and industry's growth. They even made use of it for political gain and to get a foot in the door for lucrative government contracts. But while, in theory, better equipped in terms of education, English language skills and his middle-class upbringing, Shivam's career continued to flounder, faced with hurdles and obstacles he had not expected to come in his way. His determination to change how the government as well as the public at large would perceive bodybuilding fell on deaf ears, while his involvement in various fitness-related initiatives and businesses was generally unsuccessful as well.

It is easy to argue that perhaps Shivam himself was just not cut out for his own larger-than-life ambitions. But that would be selling his story short. I believe his endeavours shed light on rural–urban entanglements and the way they colour the rapid transformation of the city's landscape in physical as well as socioeconomic terms. Caste politics, class difference and ideas of the male body and associated masculinity all impact how Shivam's individual trajectory as well as that of others unfold within this context.

## A Village Wedding in the City

A few months after we visited Bainsla's home, Shivam and I are invited to attend a wedding in a village in Greater Noida. Standing in drizzling rain next to Shivam, who is dressed in a black embroidered sherwani, we wait for the bride to exit her parental home and join her new husband in a white Mercedes that waits with the engine running. The groom is Bainsla's cousin, though I am not entirely sure about the actual family relations and neither is Shivam, for that matter. Having picked me up from the Akshardham metro station after a two-hour delay due to the heavy rains that morning, he had instructed his Ola driver to make a pit-stop at a liquor store first, explaining: 'We can't arrive sober, man, they won't like that.' The driver, who seemed somewhat intimidated by Shivam's hulking presence and thundering voice, said it would be okay for us to drink in the car but that we should keep our cups out of sight of other drivers and be vigilant for police checks. Dismissing these concerns, Shivam said: 'In these areas, cops will understand, man. We will just tell them we are headed for this wedding.' In fact, it would not surprise him if there were some politicians in attendance at the wedding. 'These people have a lot of land, money, influence, you know.'

The Ola driver dropped us somewhere on the highway from where we were picked up by an SUV that took us further afield into Greater Noida at truly breakneck speed. Racing through small villages on muddy roads lined with half-built apartments and other types of construction projects in various stages of completion, there was no escaping the ubiquitous presence of huge billboards with ads for cement companies featuring uber-muscular figures not unlike the one Shivam had sported when he took the stage himself. Recently married, he had since put on considerable weight, and confided in me that he was not working out much lately. 'All I want to lift right now is my wife!' There were also 'all these family visits to attend to', he complained, at least once every week, which left him no choice but to deviate from his diet. 'But I will be making a comeback, you will see!' A month earlier, at his wedding, I had noticed that his bride was a rather shy girl who seemed quite perplexed by Shivam's boisterousness and that of his brothers. 'But I am happy with that, you know, she won't be so demanding as my girlfriends,' he laughed, slapping my back and knocking the wind out me. 'They were always asking me for things, demanding shopping, movies, gifts.' It had exhausted him and it was also why he had agreed to this marriage proposal when it came along. 'I always say: love is for sex, arranged is for forever, no love in it.' He did not think it was necessary for this marriage to be about love. 'She comes from a poor family, but that doesn't matter to me. Her father sells shawls … They are also originally from UP, same caste, so that matters.' But the wedding we are heading to now will be very different from his own, he assured me, though the main event would have been over by the time we reach, as even the Formula One-style driving of the SUV could not make up for the considerable delay of the morning.

Shivam's own massive wedding had taken place near his house in Inderpuri, and there had also been a rather lavish engagement ceremony in Pitampura a few weeks earlier. Both times I spent most of the evening outside the venue, drinking cheap whisky from the boot of the car with Shivam's brothers and cousins while one of the waiters, who had been specially instructed, brought snacks regularly. 'You liked our food, no?' Shivam asked yet again. 'You will like the food at this wedding as well,' he assured me. 'It will be very rich though; these people really like their ghee.' It's also why they make great pehlwans he suggested. 'They have that in their blood, they're fighters these guys.' There will be no drinking from the boot of the car, though. 'You can do that in the city, but here there will be too many prying eyes. The elders won't like it.' As if reading my thoughts, Shivam explained: 'We are coming all the way from the city, so they would like us to enjoy ourselves.' And this is why we were still drinking in the car, though there was more whisky on my pants now than in the cup I was trying to bring to my mouth, thanks to the state of the road.

When we arrived, the rain had finally turned to a drizzle. Exiting the car, we crossed several courtyards, all part of the same compound that consisted of various interlinked buildings, and which was flanked by an impressive row of SUVs, until we reached an open field where we were handed paper plates with food. The groom stood next to a white Mercedes, which according to Shivam belonged to a local politician that the family had some business dealing with. He was smoking a cigarette and talking to one of his 'brothers' whom I recognised from an earlier competition. 'They are all connected, these people,' Shivam mumbled as he downed the final sip of whisky and tossed his plastic cup casually behind him. The groom also used to be a wrestler but is no longer competing, I was told.

All this information was meant to underline what Shivam had suggested earlier, that for a Gujjar family like this one, the connection with working out and 'building bodies' is a more 'natural' fit than it was for a person of Brahmin background like himself. In that sense, his own history with bodybuilding contrasts with that of Vipin and Bainsla, in that Shivam was very much a 'skinny kid' himself. 'Weak! Kamzor, we say.' One day, he got into a fight with 'this guy' from his neighbourhood who was much stronger. 'I thought, if he slaps me one more time, he will fly home without a school bus.' But he did not have the physique to follow through on this and that was his initial encouragement to start working out. Four years later, he met the same person at a local wedding and had the courage to tell him, 'Man, you better get out of my face.' Apparently, 'he could not believe himself that I had become that big'. Shivam added: 'His mind could not recognise me.' He had told his mother to make sure that 'this guy' did not come within eyesight of him again. 'By that time, I was eating twenty bananas and drinking three boxes of milk per day!' It was a memory he always recalled fondly—not just the look on the face of his former adversary but also more generally the reactions from others in his neighbourhood. His body had commanded a certain respect that it never had before. But it had also come with new questions, especially with reference to what he wanted to do with his life. He had job security but not necessarily 'job satisfaction'.

Shoes crusted with mud, the food finished and the remainder of the whisky left in the car, there is not much to do but wait for the bride to finally make it out of the house. 'Won't be long now, my man,' Shivam says. 'Patience is all there is to it.' Suddenly, a group of elderly women emerge from the house and start singing a local Gurjari song, which I am told is sung to bestow courage upon the bride as she bids farewell to her parents. Dressed in a bridal-red sari and bedecked with jewels, her face barely visible because of the veil she is carefully keeping in place, she is abundantly and 'sufficiently' overcome by grief, wailing at the top of her voice. Dryly, Shivam comments: 'She is playing her role well, man.' As the womenfolk start another song of encouragement, the bride finally gets into the car and the couple drives off. Somewhat relieved, my clothes thoroughly wet because of the rain, I discreetly ask Shivam if we can make an exit ourselves now. 'Oh no, my brother,' he says and laughs heartily, 'she will come back!' I stare at him in disbelief—'What do you mean she will come back?' Roughly ten minutes later, the car indeed returns, bride and groom in it. Barely does it come to a halt, and the bride jumps out howling. She runs to the womenfolk who had been patiently waiting, clearly expecting this to happen.

'What will happen now?'

Shivam looks surprised at this firang's odd obliviousness: 'This will happen a few more times and then we can go.' He estimates one or two times, not more. 'She can't just leave like that,' he explains. 'She needs to let her parents know how much she will miss them. That's just the way they do these things here.'

## Garlanding Gurus and Flexing Muscles

When I return to Delhi about a year later in mid-2015, I find that Shivam has decided to invest in a gym himself, and he cheerfully invites me to attend the opening. I am the first to arrive at the gym, located near Naraina Vihar metro station opposite a busy flyover in southwest Delhi. It is two o'clock in the afternoon, the time of the official opening advertised on the banner near the entrance, but no guests have arrived yet; even Shivam is stuck in traffic. As I take my seat on one of the plastic chairs that are placed in neat rows facing a temporary stage, I learn that it will likely be another hour before the first guests make an appearance. The gym is an old one, known for its local bodybuilding clientele, but no one will be let inside until the official programme wraps up. Once guests start arriving, the connection between the gym and various members of the bodybuilding federation Shivam belongs to, and whose competition he had participated in over a year earlier, becomes abundantly clear. Bainsla is there, as well as various other dignitaries such as Manosh and well-known bodybuilder and gym-owner Dinesh Aswal. The arrival of senior bodybuilder Shivkumar is met with enthusiastic applause, whistling and the vigorous shaking of hands. Once Shivam himself arrives, the official part of the programme can begin.

After a number of speeches and the garlanding of various bodybuilders and senior members of the federation, a local politician steps forward to provide Shivam with some words of wisdom, after which he asks Shivam's father to join him on stage. The two then nervously peel white shawls out from plastic wrappers which are subsequently handed out to others such as Shivkumar, who is asked to provide the audience with a bodybuilding show that he 'reluctantly' agrees to do. Quickly shedding his T-shirt, he takes the stage in his jeans and strikes various classical poses underneath the banner of the 'Hanuman Gym'. On the announcement banner, Shivam is welcomed as 'our new coach', though he basically owns it. Another banner carries the pictures of the important guests expected to be in attendance: Sh. Rajender Bainsla (Hon'ble General Secretary DBBA) ... Sh. Shiv Bainsla (Pro Body Builder, Mr Asia Gold Medallist 2013), Sh. Pradeep Bainsla (Chief Mentor Hanuman Gym).[195] Shivam's name is accompanied by the designation that he had taken fifth place in a Mr Universe competition held in Italy. Although the federation had facilitated his participation, he had paid for his own airfare and accommodation, thinking of it as an investment in his reputation as a bodybuilder and trainer.

The interaction between various dignitaries, politicians and senior bodybuilders reminds me of the many bodybuilding competitions I had attended in Delhi and elsewhere over time. In the same year as Shivam's own third place, there were various Mr Delhi competitions held across town, including one in the centrally located Talkatora Stadium. Even though it appeared to be the exact opposite of the village setting of the other competition, it was in fact organised by the same federation and the jury comprised the same members. The village elders were absent, but there was no shortage of politicians and businessmen who were called on stage to be garlanded and honoured. Non-participating bodybuilders, no matter their seniority, would head straight for the various 'gurus' in the front row and touch their feet respectfully.

Back at Shivam's grand gym opening, Shivkumar has finally been convinced, at the enthusiastic hollering of the crowd, to take off his jeans and strip down to his underwear in order to show off incredible leg muscles. His performance is followed by another bodybuilder who has been making a mark at various competitions, and finally Shivam himself. In much better shape than when we attended the wedding in Greater Noida, it is clear that his capacity 'to enjoy life' might mean he will never quite achieve the austere results showcased by Shivkumar, who has stuck to a closely monitored diet for years now and lets nothing distract him from his next workout. Having given up on his secure job, Shivam is now about to embark on an entirely new adventure. I am struck by the spartan quality of the gym that Shivam hopes will launch his career in fitness. An incredibly sober place, the equipment is old and worn though no doubt functional. As with akharas gradually doubling as gyms, catering to youngsters who no longer aspire to become wrestlers but aim to build their bodies, gyms such as this one have gradually been forced to modernise and let go of their earlier associations with the Indian model of bodybuilding.

Shivam's stint as gym manager does not last long. Within half a year, he has given up, and when I see him again in 2017, he is busy developing various business initiatives while offering personal training on the side. We meet in an office above a car showroom in Connaught Place, and I am introduced to a businessman who is involved in something called Loan Bazaar and with whom he is planning to organise a fitness event. Part of these plans include setting up his own federation, a major motivation for which is his concern that there is 'cheating' within older, established federations, especially the one he now no longer wants to be associated with. How this new federation will tackle this remains mystifyingly vague. While I too had sometimes doubted the jurors' choice of a winner now and then, I had also come to realise that the very nature of bodybuilding—with its extreme focus on the body and its relationship with the mirror—made for an inherently unstable one. Self-doubt went hand-in-hand with suspicion and paranoia, not rarely fuelled by extreme dieting and the use of controlled substances. Yet, I also knew that Shivam had never gone this far, and benefitting from 'superior genetics', as he put it, had not been known to stick to strict diets for very long.

He was also disappointed with the way 'things' had worked out with the gym so soon after his appointment as head coach and manager had been announced with so much fanfare. 'The clients were nothing there! They were just boys, sons of noodle-sellers.' As a result, he had barely made any money, even losing a considerable sum, he told me. The rant Shivam starts on does not seem to bother nor interest the businessman we are with, and who is now taking care of something on his phone. 'Bainsla really cheated me, that guy,' he repeats. Not only did he make a loss with the gym, he also found out that the federation dealt in counterfeit protein powder. Various other business plans had fallen through, one involving a piece of land and various Gujjar business partners who had squeezed him out of the deal, he claimed. 'I am not dealing with these people, anymore!' He then declared, 'We are high-class Brahmin people!'

## WRESTLING WITH BODYBUILDING

In 2014, Indian as well as international media briefly flocked to the village of Asola-Fatehpur Beri, which lies halfway between Gurgaon and Faridabad towards Haryana's border. With only 3,500 inhabitants, there is little about the village that is remarkable other than the fact that about 90 per cent of its men between the ages of eighteen and fifty-five work as bouncers and security guards in Delhi. A short report online shows local men working out with weights, not unlike the way they would in ordinary gyms, even though their diets are rooted in pehlwani wrestling.[196] The name of the head trainer, Vijay Pahelwan, underscores this connection. He recommends three to four litres of milk per day as well as a dozen bananas and half a kilo of chiku.[197] In *Enter the Dangal: Travels through India's Wrestling Landscape*, sports journalist R. Sengupta (2016) describes the diet of one of the wrestling champions he has been following in similar terms: 'Satbir ... eats his way through roughly a quarter of a kilo each of almonds, dal and paneer, half a kilo each of fruits and vegetables, a kilo of milk ...'[198] Even though this wrestler also makes use of 'US-made protein powder and vitamin supplements', his diet would never result in the desired muscularity, leanness and vascularity in order to be competitive on a bodybuilding stage. Yet, for the profession of bouncer or security guard, it will easily endow these men with the kind of bulkiness required to intimidate.

While the growing demand for bouncers and security guards is linked to India's recent economic growth and new middle-class formations, these professions offer decidedly less opportunities for socioeconomic mobility than that of a personal trainer, with its often intimate relationship between client and trainer. In that sense, these 'village bodies' resonate with an earlier masculine ideal of strength and might, but are less impressive in terms of the 'knowledge' that has gone into crafting them—a fact that is underlined by the trainers' repeated stress on their own expertise and scientific grasp of the arc of transformation. It is typically 'merely' a body that intimidates. Vipin, with his typical (former) pehlwani physique, moved to South Delhi not just to adopt a different type of workout routine and dietary regimen under the guidance of Bainsla, but also to put physical distance between himself and his village. Even though his extended family is relatively well-off, making it into bodybuilding and offering personal training to well-off Delhiites, he reasoned, would provide him with purpose and perhaps even the means to sustain himself and provide for his family independently.

Delhi's ambitions to become a world-class city are clearly infused with the notion of it as a place of upward mobility, both in terms of what the city has to offer as well as what it facilitates: economic growth, new opportunities for leisure and consumption, and a buzzing business climate that guarantees the city's competitiveness. Delhi is now India's largest city and may one day even represent the largest urban agglomeration in the world. This does not only mean a changing urban landscape that is 'engulfing villages' in its wake, but also increasing diversity in terms of who considers the city 'home'. The cases of Shivam, Bainsla, Vipin and other members of the Gujjar-dominated bodybuilding federation discussed provide a glimpse into the changing dynamics and power hierarchies as they give shape to trajectories of upward socioeconomic mobility. By nature, these trajectories are unfinished, ongoing and, like the city itself, under construction. As enduring and strong as the quality of concrete that is advertised on giant billboards across the NCR may be, middle-class lives are far from set in stone, their foundations are constantly challenged and its flexibility tested.

Within Delhi the relationship between village and city identities is clearly dichotomous and adversarial. However, they are dichotomous mainly in the imagination and as a tool to make sense of a rapidly changing urban environment. What stands out in Joseph Alter's seminal work on pehlwani wrestling is that his informants clearly distinguish their own practices from those of bodybuilders. The dyad informing this also guides the distinction between bodybuilding and most other types of sport. The focus in bodybuilding is principally on the exterior, whereas the wrestler takes a more holistic and 'internal' approach here. For a pehlwan, his body is not just one that is developed keeping victory in the wrestling pit in mind, but also one that constitutes a lifestyle that extends beyond working out and strict diets. Yet, within Delhi-based gyms, the wrestler's body was rarely appreciated. The association with village backgrounds, rural masculinities and the potential of encountering 'such men' as 'rowdy types' and 'who make their living as bouncers', sets wrestlers apart from the trainers that clients encounter in the gym. The latter are men they trust with providing guidance in terms of workout routines and diets, and who would often even function as lifestyle coaches. But it is clear that the relationship between client and trainer remains paradoxical. While they were well regarded within the gym and trusted for their 'knowledge', outside these men's rural backgrounds and caste identities would be cause for concern and suspicion. As rapidly as the city might be changing, these pre-held notions were made of decidedly sturdy material.

# CHAPTER 6

# SEX & DESIRE

*But the expression of a well-made man appears not only in
his face,*
*It is in his limbs and joints also, it is curiously in the joints of
his hips and wrists,*
*It is in his walk, the carriage of his neck, the flex of his waist
and knees, dress does not hide him…*

— Walt Whitman[199]

As Raj takes a shower, streams of water snaking down his
sculpted chest, it is clear that his mind is preoccupied.
The movie is quick to reveal why—memories of a joyful time
spent with his girlfriend alternate with flashbacks of a romantic
and passionate encounter with a male friend named Aryan. The
camera focuses languidly on Raj's hand caressing his abdominal
muscles, allowing the viewer to contemplate the predicament he
must be in. This is the opening scene of a YouTube production
called *Other Side of Love*—announced as a 'gay-themed Hindi
Bollywood Suspense Thriller Drama Film'—directed, produced
and written by Ambrish Bhatia. The scene continues with Aryan

approaching Raj from behind and placing his hands on Raj's chest. Raj turns around swiftly and angrily demands to know what he thinks he's doing. Aryan retorts that he is doing this because of 'love'. Referring to Raj's girlfriend, he says: 'She is not at home, that's why I have come.' Returning his hands to Raj's wet chest, he says: 'it feels pleasurable to bathe with you ... looks like these water droplets are burning after falling on your body.' Bringing a wet finger to his lips, he adds: 'And I feel to touch these burning water droplets to my body to satisfy my inner self.' Raj then pushes him away, saying, 'I'll sue you in a minute.' But his friend is unimpressed and pulls him closer, pressing upon him that this is exactly what he wants: 'I want you to turn wild because I love wild men.'

The men speak in Hindi, but there is a point to using the clumsy translation of the movie subtitles here. It is revealing for the context from which this movie has emerged and its imagined audience. The filmmaker, Ambrish Bhatia, is a chain-smoking elderly man in his sixties, and a software and website developer by day. He is well known in fitness circles for his photography and videography of muscular adolescent men, and his following on Facebook and YouTube has rapidly increased over the years. I first learned of his work when his photographs started gaining traction on social media around 2013. Invariably shot in heritage sites such as forts and palaces, most of his photoshoots are meant to look like they had been conducted as part of a joyful road trip. Even though the occasional girl is included as well, the vast majority are of young men, some still dealing with acne, and featured bare-chested in jeans or underwear, seductively gazing into the camera and flaunting their sculpted physiques. The idea behind these photoshoots as well as later video projects is to provide a platform for local youth from Faridabad and the surrounding areas to showcase their potential as models and to secure contracts for professional assignments. Yet, Bhatia's work is also undeniably homoerotic, and shot in a manner that feels excessive and convoluted. While he is indeed presenting these men with a platform for 'local talent', offering them the opportunity to garner experience and build a portfolio, the entrenched homoeroticism of his work—and the way same-sex desire features prominently in his video projects—also raises questions about who the audience for his work truly is.

In *Other Side of Love*, both Aryan and Raj are highly skilled professionals. Raj is the head of a marketing department and Aryan a software engineer recruited to help him secure an important business deal. The third role is performed by the only woman in the movie, Neha, who is the HR manager of a competing company, of which Ambrish Bhatia himself plays the general manager. While Neha also happens to be Raj's girlfriend, from the moment Raj and Aryan shake hands, there is an intense, brooding energy between the two. A scene, which depicts Aryan lustfully observing Raj removing his shirt in the hotel room that they share on a business trip, underlines this. That evening, they make love, but when the next morning Aryan professes he has fallen in love with Raj and cannot live without him, the latter brushes this off, telling him not to be 'too clingy' and that he has a long list of lovers. The story then quickly turns soap opera-esque, with bewildering plot-turns involving a fourth character named Vicky who is after the same business deal. Neha, we learn, actually has a 'village connection' with Aryan, and is mainly out to teach Raj a lesson because he had an affair with her brother who has been unconscious ever since. While it remains unclear what exactly transpired between the two—we only learn that Raj fulfilled her brother's desires and then left him in a state of coma—the movie's subtext appears to be that there is something innately deceitful and dangerous about same-sex desire and homosexual relationships. The fact that Aryan has stored evidence of his encounter with Raj on his laptop underscores this, a problem that Vicky offers to solve with 'a hot boy' who will sleep with Aryan (for which he has an alleged 'weakness'). Meanwhile, the plan is for Vicky to access Aryan's laptop and phone to delete the incriminating evidence. Somewhere down the line, it turns out that it was actually Neha's idea to blackmail Raj. She had him followed by a detective, who made the video, which she subsequently asks Aryan to confront her boyfriend with. Eventually, all differences are settled and we are left with a somewhat happy ending in which Neha and Raj are reunited, the former content with the lesson she taught her lover. Even though cordial relations are restored, Aryan bids them farewell, moving elsewhere altogether. The danger of same-sex desire has been vanquished, and no longer poses a threat to the heterosexual relationship that Neha and Raj are now left to enjoy in peace—thus putting a 'straightjacket' on Raj's sculpted body, which Aryan had desired so forcefully.

There is a complexity obliquely embedded in Ambrish Bhatia's work, freely available on YouTube: while on the one hand there is the lingering gaze resting casually on the male body, exploring and navigating its muscular beauty, on the other, the various storylines point at the pitfalls of male modelling itself, warning against the risk of abuse and exploitation, and ultimately pointing at the assumed inherent duplicity of homoerotic desire. Bhatia claims that the movies are based on his numerous interactions with young aspiring male models. So are these movies the 'truth' as he sees it? Or are they themselves evidence of a particular urban fantasy? If this is what is being imagined, what does it build on? In all my years of research, I have only come across one trainer who is now actually involved in escort work. This does not mean, of course, that others do not capitalise on the sexual desire their bodies radiate. In fact, the tagging and descriptions on social media often explicitly capture their bodies as being sexually attractive. However, sex itself—whether with women or men—remained paradoxically absent from narratives throughout. The personal history of Selvam, who does provide sexual services and is involved in pornographic activities, provides an entry point to understand how class impacts the way sexual desire is interpreted, regulated and acted upon in urban India.

## THE ABSENCE AND PRESENCE OF SEXUAL DESIRE

One evening in Chennai, I am catching up with personal trainer Selvam. In his early thirties, he is a strikingly handsome man with clear movie-star potential. Involved in regular photoshoots across India, he generously shares the results with his ballooning following on Instagram. I compliment him on a recent photoshoot with 'Man of Madras', a photographic platform mainly operating on Instagram that somewhat exclusively works with Tamil models, and ask if he has ever considered a career in acting. He brusquely dismisses the very possibility. 'I would need so many connections …' Considering his impoverished background, 'that just wouldn't work', he said. 'It's not a system based on talent. Or not purely on talent … I have to live with the chances that I have been given,' he adds contemplatively. He has just ordered a mocktail and what he determines to be the healthiest meal on the menu: herb-coated chicken breast and lots of vegetables. He is unfamiliar with the 'French' preparation but keen to try it out, as he is with most things in life, he professes. Even if most of his photoshoots take place in lush and luxurious locations, such as in and around the swimming pools of five-star properties or inside posh hotel bedrooms—where he does things like seductively stepping out of a shower stall with a bathrobe barely covering his private parts—Selvam admits that it's a world still by and large alien to him. Now providing sexual services to affluent male customers and selling pornographic videos on websites such as *Only Fans*, his career has taken a direction that is the stuff of urban fantasies.

For men with bodies that are presented as patently sexually attractive in popular media, and that trainers and bodybuilders often hashtag with #hotbody and #sexybeast on social media, it is remarkable how absent sex was from their accounts of day-to-day life. This contrasted rather amusingly with the way gay friends pulled my leg, suggesting that I had opportunistically located my research in a candy store with the owner absent and the laddoos up for grabs. Jat-men especially were always up for it, I was once assured, 'not even necessarily for money', as my friend put it. In fact, Malayali men too could be easily had, I was told; well-hung, physically strong and muscular—'they are quite the meat eaters, you know'—and most important of all, not perturbed by same-sex contact. 'It doesn't mean much to them,' an acquaintance from Bangalore had declared. 'They don't think of it as an issue.' Questions from academic audiences aligned with the impression that fitness instructors, especially those from intermediate castes, were easily available for sexual encounters, whether of the straight or same-sex variety. For instance, I would frequently be asked whether these men were involved in sex work, or at the very least preyed upon by female clients for sexual services. Invariably, such questions would come with the disclaimer that it was not something the questioners themselves were interested in, but something they had wondered about, having observed 'such men' in the gym. Rumours clearly abounded!

I once asked a female academic colleague from Delhi where she had gotten the idea that fitness trainers were easily available for sexual services. She replied with a dismissive shrug: 'It's out there.' What was fuelling this idea? What exactly was 'out there'? And how could it be that it only played such a marginal role in my discussions with trainers and bodybuilders, some of whom I had known for years? I had met their families, knew their wives, interacted with their parents, celebrated religious occasions together, and had frequently been the listening ear to deeply held anxieties about financial worries, bodily insecurities and the potentially debilitating side effects of controlled substances. The idea that these men were available for sexual adventures clearly contrasted with the reaction of trainers and bodybuilders themselves; they either said 'such things' simply did not happen in their gyms or were puzzled by what I was implying in the first place. The gym was held to be a 'straight' and straight-forward place; to question the gaze that dawdles on a body in the process of working out or posing in front of the mirror challenges what is held to be a desexualised space. Within this space, male trainers were permitted to touch their female clients to adjust their postures, while male clients were able to pose bare chested in front of the mirror with these very same female clients continuing their workout, seemingly unperturbed. To assume otherwise not only sexualised a safe space—something that was also explicitly part of the training and guidelines provided to new hires—but also breached the perceived boundaries that separated clients and trainers.

Class difference is not just crucial to understanding what informs such boundaries between clients and trainers but also interpretations of sexual desire, desirability and availability. While the possibility of upward social mobility is an important reason why the profession of fitness trainer has gradually gained in popularity among lower-middle-class men, the potential of sexual intimacy and longer-term relationships are not on the horizon. Ambrish Bhatia's movies attempt to caution young, lower-middle-class Indians about the pitfalls of male modelling and the potentially exploitative intentions of gay men. He also seems to point to the risks involved in transgressing middle-class boundaries. In his vision, attractive, naïve, adolescent men are up for grabs by those more at home in a rapidly changing urban India—an India that cares nothing for old norms. Even though it remains in question what Bhatia's own motivations are, his take on the matter does align with accounts of trainers and bodybuilders and their forays into modelling. The jocular exuberance of some of my gay friends certainly confirmed that 'these men' were preyed upon and considered 'easy kill'. While most trainers and bodybuilders considered the gym a place of work, for my friends, these sites made for alarmingly red dots on an imaginary map of sexual debauchery. Sex was everywhere, in the polite but timid smile of an attractive personal trainer, the gentle correcting touch of a hot yoga instructor, or the determined and masculine instructions of a handsome bodybuilder whose coy smile betrayed his softer (naïve, provincial, small town) nature. In their experience, this was an integral aspect of attending and hanging out in gyms, perhaps even its most important lure. They told me that the steam and locker rooms provide bountiful opportunities for same-sex encounters. Trainers might share their phone number for off-hours interaction, the anonymity of the spa made 'hungry' groping possible, and of course there was always the possibility of house-calls. Oh, the sheer glee of all there was to see and sample!

## From Modelling to Sex Work

There is no denying the abundance of cruising spaces and the possibilities for same-sex encounters in India, but there was a striking mismatch between what my friends assumed to be possible and happening, and the everyday accounts trainers and bodybuilders shared me with me over time. The slantwise homoerotic quality of some informants' social media updates contrasted with their own accounts as well, though. When I brought this up during interviews—frolicking around on a beach in Kerala, their bodies seductively smeared with sand, wearing a tiny pair of swimming trunks from a brand such as Andrew Christian and Aussiebum (popular among gay men)— the rationale was that such pictures brought out the strength and muscular qualities of their bodies. These photoshoots were meant to secure lucrative modelling contracts that could supplement their income as fitness trainers, raise their demand among high-end clients, and help finance their trajectories as bodybuilders. In fact, informants would pay considerable amounts for such photoshoots in the hope of such gains. Even if the photographer had waived his usual fee with the idea that the photos might strengthen his own portfolio as a fashion photographer, the flight to and stay in an exotic location would still mean a considerable investment on the part of the aspiring model. However, these men did need to navigate the inherent homoeroticism that imbued these photoshoots. The complaints that they felt preyed upon by photographers and Bollywood representatives, who offered to assist them in return for sexual favours, indicated that their own desirability among members of the same sex frequently presented itself as something to be dealt with.

I had initially come across Selvam's pictures because of his collaborations with photographers whose work seemed to be gaining traction among some of my informants. Like with Ambrish Bhatia's initial photography work, their output aligned with a certain homoerotic aesthetic. How did these pictures appear to appeal to such different registers of desire? At one level there was the pure and unadulterated appreciation of a fitness- and bodybuilding-oriented crowd, at another level there were the lurid comments not rarely accompanied by love-struck smileys and eggplant emoticons. Unlike other informants, Selvam's updates directly appealed to a gay audience in terms of how he could fulfil their wildest imaginations. Who was this man who was confident enough to put himself out there in this way? When I initially approached Selvam via Instagram, he responded rather quickly by describing himself as 'basically a gym trainer' who had 'started other side jobs like fitness modelling to top up [his] salary'. Our conversation—initially via Instagram and WhatsApp—quickly turned quite insightful about why a trainer would sell his body. Yet, even more so, Selvam's story highlights the complex interplay of socioeconomic factors that ultimately govern the way a 'beautiful body' like his own might get appropriated, used and even abused for the very reason of assumed accessibility.

Back in the bar in Chennai, Selvam looks tired. He has come straight from the airport after finishing a video-shoot in Mumbai for his *Only Fans* account. The way he usually organises such shoots is by finding a trainer who would be willing to have sex with him on camera. His participation in bodybuilding and fitness-modelling competitions are also oriented towards this. Selvam knows that he does not necessarily have it in him to be competitive on stage, but such events brimmed with an abundance in terms of recruiting 'new talent', as he put it. 'Many of these guys are in need of money, and salaries in gyms are not so high, so that may convince them.' He is surely not the only one who, on top of financing his own fitness ambitions, has to support a family back home. How far a video would go greatly depends on the person he works with—from a simple 'barely explicit' shower scene, where they would both lather each other with soap and then rinse off, to oral sex or even anal penetration and group sex. He considers himself 'basically straight who became bisexual due to exposure', by which he means that when he began with fitness modelling, 'some photographers wanted to have sex with me'. Social media followers would soon approach him for the same. 'Now we all kinda know this might happen,' he says. 'So we take it lightly. Just close your eyes and let your dick be sucked. A mouth is a mouth at the end of the day.'

He now regularly travels to other cities, such as Bangalore, where he performs as a go-go dancer at gay parties held at a posh five-star hotel. These are parties where he dances on stage, even though he had no idea how to dance, he says with a smirk. 'Just go with the flow, I thought.' Selvam got involved with go-go dancing through his Instagram profile: 'They had two models and needed a third one, so I just took the offer.' For one evening of work, he was paid Rs 10,000 plus accommodation, which he considered a handsome sum. But the prime motivator was what it may generate in the long run. 'It's a great place to scout for future clients.' If he decides to sleep with a client, his charges depend on the requirements. 'It can go from six-K till twenty-K.' Requirements can vary in terms of 'duration, soft/hard role etc'. But there are always those who try to bargain and 'who want to pay you three-K'. About this he is very clear: 'God bless the "block" button ... I mean, with all due respect, if you don't have money, don't waste it on escorts.' It's a service for people with 'extra available incomes', he opines, adding that he delivers quality and that comes with a price tag.

## JUST REMOVE YOUR CLOTHES

The first time Selvam got involved in sex work was through a photographer who had contacted him for a shoot. 'He said one client from Dubai likes Indian guys very much and he wants to meet me to see and touch my body.' It was clear that he would pay well, though he doesn't remember the exact amount. Selvam agreed and went to meet this client at his hotel. 'Just remove my clothes and flex my muscles, etc. He touched my body and jerked off.' He describes the experience as 'very OK'. He didn't know that this was something he would be doing beforehand though. But he was okay with the situation since it was not very invasive. 'I didn't have to do anything.' But surely the social stigma must have crossed his mind? Boldly, Selvam responds: 'For me, I just think someone is enjoying my body.' He goes even further and asks: 'What's the point of having a hot body if you cannot enjoy or make others enjoy? It's not going to be a museum piece!'

In the course of our conversations, however, it becomes clear that his boldness is something of a façade, thinly veiling a rather painful family history that has contributed to his current position. Growing up in a small village outside Chennai—which he describes as the 'one-shop variety'—he used to work at a small grocery store from six o'clock till nine o'clock in the morning while completing his tenth standard in school. After that there was no more money and he left school altogether. His eloquence in English is, therefore, mainly the result of self-study. He once put this as 'I am a pakka village guy', something which struck him as fairly hilarious considering where he was now. Most of his English he learned via YouTube. 'I watched all the videos for English grammar and all that ... There are so many videos. It's very easy. Just watch a couple of videos every day.' Initially, the family had some money, but his father was a 'useless alcoholic' and there were always any number of bills to be paid. As a result, 'there was only money to educate one child, so they decided to educate my sister'. The reason for this was that 'she was much elder to me and she could start working sooner and support the family'. While his sister studied for her MBBS to become a doctor, Selvam 'went to work on the fields'.

When the time came to marry off his sister, the search for a suitable husband began. In due course, a groom, who seemed to tick all boxes in terms of caste and education, was found. However, the day before the wedding, there was a fight between his sister and her fiancé. 'Some nasty words were said', and the wedding was cancelled. 'My sister couldn't take it. She managed to get a bottle of poison and killed herself.' It left the family devastated. 'All our savings and assets were invested in her', with the promise that she would start working and start supporting the family. Now the family had lost everything. 'Dowry was just the last savings. After that we were left with nothing.' But it wasn't only about the money. 'I really loved my sister. She was like a hero to me. The one who was refined and educated.' She was the one who could speak English, who was intelligent, Selvam continued. 'But nobody knew of the demons that were nesting in her heart.'

With the family's loans mounting, Selvam decided to head to Chennai to make money there. He slept on the streets while searching for employment, which he eventually found with a team that catered at weddings, for which he was paid Rs 90 a day. He would make roughly Rs 1,800 per month, of which he would send Rs 600 to his mother. He then found employment as a security guard, which paid marginally better at Rs 2,200 per month. Quite by chance, he found a large sum of money in a temple, which a worshipper had accidentally left behind. When he returned the money, he was awarded a job as a supervisor with a construction company out of gratitude. He stayed there for nearly ten years. Meanwhile, he had become 'very focused' on his body and had started working out regularly. His 'good looks', as he put it himself, had already told him that there was money to be made with it, though perhaps not in the most conventional way. Living on the streets of Chennai, he would sometimes get picked up by men who would want to have sex with him. Realising his body's potential, he had also taken to visiting a local cruising site where he would occasionally make 'some money'. It was eventually through his first attempt at landing a 'modelling gig' that he realised that his body would always evoke this kind of desire and that he may as well capitalise on it.

## The Soft Look or What 'Exactly' Appeals

Selvam's difficult story aligns with that of other trainers in terms of the predicaments that trajectories of upward socioeconomic mobility may come with, and the way the body can be used as currency in this. It reminded me of a conversation I once had with Girish,[200] a bodybuilder from North Delhi who had made no secret of his own modelling ambitions. Frequently updating his social media accounts, on which he had thousands of followers, with photographs of himself in the latest branded underwear and swimwear, he seemed well aware of his good looks beyond the immediate appeal of his muscular body. The comments following one of the pictures in which he had lifted up his shirt and pulled down his jogging pants far enough not only to reveal his highly defined abs but also the veins which suggestively snaked down to his crotch, had varied from the rudimentary pictorial thumbs-ups to far more sexually laced ones. He never read those, he said: 'I don't really have time for that.' Indiscriminately though, he would provide them with a *like*, saying that he was grateful that people took the time to comment and seemed to appreciate the hard work he had put into his body.

When we met at a Starbucks outlet in Pitampura (North Delhi) one day, heads craned to size him up and conversations abruptly ended. Wearing a white polo, the sleeves of which were barely able to cover his protruding biceps, dinner-plate sized pectoral muscles pushing through the fabric revealing a muscular cleavage, he was clearly a sight to behold. Girish had spent the morning in the gym and was now on a break, which he usually used to sleep in order to be fit enough for his evening workout. Shyly, he explained that his main goal now was 'to become bigger' in order to be competitive in the next weight class, but he was worried that this might make him less appealing for future modelling assignments. 'They don't like it when we get too big.' In fact, this was something he had been told when some recruiters had approached him for a possible campaign a few months earlier as well. The money coming in through personal training was not nearly enough to compensate for the investment he was making in his body in terms of protein powders, supplements, steroids and growth hormones, something for which he continued to rely on family for support. Modelling would provide a welcome additional income, but he had been put off by the requests for sexual favours. 'I am not a gay,' he explained. 'Some go for that,' meaning other models, 'but it's not for me.'

It was a sentiment personal trainer and aspiring model Bikram also voiced when I interviewed him in relation to a recent photoshoot that I had come across on social media. In it, he is seen cavorting on a beach in Goa, his precision-engineered body covered with streaks of sand, a pair of tiny red swimming pants leaving little to the imagination. The pictures conveyed utter confidence in his body and himself. The videos he regularly uploaded on his YouTube channel, and which he readily shared on Facebook to a steadily growing audience, underlined this confidence, particularly in the malleability of the male body and what could be achieved with it. Having arrived in Delhi seven years earlier, he had gradually transitioned from providing fitness and personal training in gyms to 'online coaching' with clients mainly based abroad. In search of alternatives to taking 'drugs' to build his body, he had at some point come across a link to MuscleMania, a drug-free competition for natural bodybuilders, which had immediately appealed to him. And because Bollywood was a dream in the back of his mind, Bikram decided to compete in the Mumbai event instead of the one in Delhi, where he was based. By that time, various Bollywood recruiters had already contacted him, but he had come to realise that '90 per cent of these are fake'. They will suggest developing a portfolio for which 'they ask you to pay', but 'that's the way they make their money'. Meanwhile, Bollywood was also not necessarily his biggest dream, as he put it. 'I wanted to transform fitness.' The transformation of his own body, without the use of steroids or hormones, was key to this plan. Sharing his transformation and various wins in bodybuilding competitions via social media was paying off. 'Some see me as their inspiration and motivation.' And as a result: 'they go to the gym 'cause of me'. A growing number of photoshoot requests followed. 'Now I have fans abroad, they comment on my pictures all the time.' A girl in the US even has his poster above her bed. 'She said so, that she had used one of my pictures to make a poster. This feeling left me so much proud.'

During a long conversation, Bikram mentioned that he received 'lots of messages from gays'. Some of these concerned offers for Bollywood parts, 'but I don't know if it's right'. Contemplating this, he added: 'I know one-two things ...' He said he had some friends in Bollywood whom he utilised as a sounding board to double-check the kind of invitations and requests he received. 'They warned me for that. These people might take your money, more.' He was even contacted by a US-based porn star who wanted to do a video with him. She performs live on camera, so he knew she was 'the real deal'. He had clearly done his research. The porn star in question offered him $1,200 to star in a video, but in the end he did not follow through on the plan. Now that he has some experience with modelling, he is particularly keen to work with beginners. 'I tell them to do something different.' One of these young photographers did his Goa shoot. 'They are not from rich parents, these guys.' When they did the shoot in Goa, he paid for his own flight and accommodation, which cost him around Rs 25,000. But he felt it was worth it since it had led to other opportunities, such as one where he had been asked to model for Aussiebum, a deal that eventually did not work out for reasons he did not explain.

About the shape and form of his body, he is quite specific. 'I don't want to become a bulky bodybuilder.' Bikram aims 'to look handsome and sexy'. What he has in mind is for his clients to say: 'This kind of body looks good, that's what we like.' As such, he 'believes in aesthetics'. Even if he was in the process of 'putting on weight' to later convert this into additional muscle for the next season, he emphasises that he does not want to overdo it: 'I want to go for that soft look.' This is different from what bodybuilders go for, he once assured me. 'They want that hard look, muscles and veins'—not what modelling recruiters are interested in. 'I have that balanced body; the fashion industry—they like that.' He likes that they sometimes get confused about where he is from. 'Sometimes they say Latin, other times Burmese.' It makes him mysterious, he feels. 'But always they wonder, how did he change himself?'

## To Go Fully Bold and Never Say No

In 2014, I met Ambrish Bhatia at his house in Faridabad, which doubled as his studio and functioned as a hangout for the kind of adolescent men who are central to his various projects. Quick to point out that he was first and foremost a software developer,

Ambrish explained that he only considered the modelling photography 'a starting profession' for himself, meaning that he thought of himself as a beginner. That said, within a relatively short time he had developed a considerable online and offline following of aspiring models, mainly hailing from the NCR. Most had established contact through Facebook or referral, as he put it. 'They contact me that way. They contact me and then come down.' Browsing through his computer while lighting a cigarette, he mentioned that a shoot he had recently completed was with six boys and one girl. 'They are not friends, they don't know each other.' The only person they had in common was Ambrish himself. 'I arrange the group events and then I do the group shoots.' In selecting potential candidates for his projects, he emphasised that the figure is not his main criterion. With reference to a photoshoot that had taken place the previous day, and of which he had shown me unedited pictures, he suggested that his main interests are style and expression. 'I don't focus much on the body.' He tapped the screen with a nicotine-stained finger to underline his point. 'Attitude is more important, as well as style.' However, when I mentioned that most of his work seemed quite focused on the physique of his male models, he admitted that 'the figures are there, sure, some have good figures'. With a couple of clicks of his mouse, he showed me a young man lying on a tree trunk in nothing but the tiniest red posing trunk, seductively looking into the camera, his muscular body on full display. 'Not many have that body though. They have the expressions but not that body. We use that.'

At the time, Ambrish was yet to embark on his video project, the 2014 movie *Marichika*, which is described as a 'Gay Themed Hindi Short Film on Exploitation of Gay Models'. The movie, which runs for about forty-five minutes, commences with two adolescent men casually hanging out on a boat on the river with some Mughal heritage buildings as a backdrop. They are discussing what it takes to make dreams come true, something that is clearly on the mind of the protagonist. He confides in his friend that he may run away to Delhi and pursue his dream of becoming a model instead of joining the family business. His friend is quick to support him and offers to introduce him to a Delhi-based acquaintance (Anish) who is into modelling himself. When they meet not much later, Anish immediately suggests that good looks are not enough, and that it also takes style, attitude and boldness. Since the aspiring model is from a village, he may need some help with this, which leads Anish to ask what he is willing to do to become a model. The response is 'anything', to which Anish retorts: 'Anything means a lot in this world.'[201] First of all, he will have to change his lifestyle. 'Fully Bold!!! You should never say NO for anything.' After some sessions in the gym, he is also informed that he needs a portfolio for which he will have to arrange a photoshoot which may cost him about Rs 20–25,000. However, Anish has a friend who may be able to make this work for as little as Rs 10–15,000. It leads the main character to take out a loan on a 20 per cent interest rate. With the stage set for potential abuse, we witness how a casting director asks him to strip during a session and subsequently manages to sleep with him. As the story unfolds, we realise that he has done this to others as well, but that there are also honourable men in the business who will not take advantage of a beginner model's precarious financial situation. As the movie comes to a close, a final warning is offered: 'People will exploit you, if you are ready to get exploited.'

The understanding that those involved in India's male fashion industry run a considerable risk of exploitation is confirmed in a long piece that appeared in the magazine *Open*, in which

Shefalee Vasudev investigates the world of male models in India.[202] While there is substantial demand for female models, it is much more limited for their male counterparts. As the president of the Fashion Design Council of India (FDCI) put it, only 5 per cent of the shows that are held as part of Amazon India Fashion Week include menswear.[203] Besides, menswear brands tend to prefer film celebrities and sport stars.[204] Accordingly, in India's smaller towns, male models work for anything between Rs 2,000 and Rs 6,000 per assignment, which could be as long as two days. Male models get only a quarter of what female models are paid.[205] Sexual favours turn out to be common, as Arry Dabas, a winner of various modelling titles, reveals. Dabas suggests that because of the combination of good looks, great bodies and sex appeal, they are automatic objects of desire. 'We are trophies, to be given away in the bedroom, a benchmark of attainment for power brokers.'[206] Furthermore, unregistered model coordinators who act as event managers are known to abuse young aspirants, making them work without pay, even sending them out to parties with open-ended possibilities. The comments of one brand director are revealing. He notes that a good body itself does not make for a good model, 'as scores of boys from small towns seem to believe'. What is also necessary are 'good manners, personality, grooming and educational background'[207] as well as the ability to make the 'right decision'. The willingness to become models—even if the total package does not add up in terms of the body, its dimensions and additional prerequisites—thus becomes one of desperation if we approach it from the logic of socioeconomic difference, understood from the perspective of all those in the know about what is required 'besides' a good body.

While the characters portrayed in Ambrish Bhatia's movies are generally highly skilled professionals and businessmen, the actors speak in Hindi and appear to be portraying an aspiration rather than something they are actually familiar with. The subtitles too betray an ambivalent relationship with the English language, something that the comments section underlines as well. The videos clearly cater to adolescent men of similar backgrounds, and appeal to their desire to act and learn more about opportunities in modelling. Bhatia's own goals are somewhat mystifying here. Over the years, I have attempted to discuss this with him, but he constantly emphasises that his involvement is mainly about making sure that male models are prepared for what awaits them.

His concerns are not limited to exploitation by conmen and gatekeepers in the industry but also by what young models themselves might be willing to provide in exchange for favours. During our conversation in Faridabad in 2014, Bhatia provided me with the example of a model named Vikas who had recently requested Ambrish to shoot him naked. 'But I am not giving! I am not into that!' Apparently, this aspiring model had made acquaintance with a person in Australia who had offered him Rs 15,000 if he did the shoot naked. He had sought Ambrish's advice, and he had told him, 'No. Don't do it.' Most men who had made similar requests over time had wanted 'these photos to flatter themselves', desiring 'to present themselves in the glamour world'. He assured me it was 'clicks' they were after, meaning likes on social media. Given that he's a straight-identified man with a wife and children himself, why does Ambrish often insert gay themes in his movies? I asked him that question, and he answered: 'No, it is not like this, it's the concept which I get in mind.' For this he took inspiration from the many stories that had been shared with him about male modelling, he said. His actors were never uncomfortable with depicting same-sex attraction or relations, he assured me, 'because I teach them that an actor is one who can play any character, and in my last movie, I played myself as a gay father.' None of the actors he had worked with were gay themselves, he said, and added: 'few are students, few are doing business', as if to underline that it was not a genuine possibility that they were homosexual.

## Sexual Capital of the Male Body

Desire and desirability are crucial elements in understanding what produces the lean, muscular body in the gym as well as the way it is imagined, represented and depicted outside. There is something incontrovertible about how building, developing and working on the body is layered with an interplay of desire and desirability. The scripted adulation around the bodily transformation of male heroes in Indian movies is imbued with a homoeroticism that has often been explained in terms of the relatively limited possibilities for sexual contact between members of the opposite sex in India and the strength of male friendships. The argument is that this may also explain same-sex contact between adolescent Indian men who do not necessarily identify as gay or question their sexual identity because of same-sex attraction. However, this explanation does not adequately consider the manner in which class difference factors into the way same-sex contact and desire operate and are negotiated in India. Male friendship is often captured as 'dosti', a Hindi descriptor that has gradually come to denote a whole interplay of notions such as camaraderie, companionship and closeness among men, describing an imaginary spectrum from holding hands in public as a sign of affection to same-sex contact in the absence of access to members of the other sex. The use of the word 'mast(i)', on the other hand, comes with a tinge of sexual flavour, naughtiness, casualness, taking on a sexualised fun quotient. While a movie can be mast, or a particular actor can look mast, masti friendships may also involve same-sex contact, though primarily understood as a temporary phase characteristic of adolescent years. Increasingly, such notions of dosti and masti have come to reflect socioeconomic difference because this type of male friendship and intimacy has been downgraded to exclusively reference working or lower-middle-class 'vernac' relations between adolescent men.[208] This is then held to contrast with relations between English-speaking upper-middle-class men who would, for instance, not consider holding hands because of its 'globalised' association with same-sex identities.

Bollywood, therefore, treads a precarious balance, and it is not always easy to understand the specific intention of a movie's homoerotic undertones. A Delhi-based friend had once slyly remarked about this: 'It kind of depends what you read into it.' A rare example of a hit movie that does acknowledge the homoerotic potential of the male body is *Dostana* (2008), even if it does not necessarily take seriously the potential for same-sex relations. Homoerotic innuendo and same-sex desire mark more recent movies, such as *Gunday* (2014) and *Padmaavat* (2018), even if their storylines ultimately revolve around a desirable woman. In an article for *Firstpost*, author Deepanjana Pal hilariously captures what is truly at stake in the movie *Gunday*.[209] Although it was released on Valentine's Day, this action flick is perhaps not an automatic romantic choice. However, as Pal puts it, 'the way Ranveer Singh and Arjun

Kapoor bared their cleavages and looked into each other's eyes in the trailer', many deduced 'that there was bromance broiling under *Gunday's* macho surface'. Pal even typifies the movie as a love story 'of two men whom heterosexuality—as embodied by Priyanka Chopra—tries to separate'. The characters Singh and Kapoor depict, therefore, make for an ideal couple: 'they run together, they dance with each other, they mud wrestle without breaking eye contact, they can communicate with one another without words'. In fact, Pal even argues that the character portrayed by Ranveer Singh 'flounces his hair the way heroines have for decades in Bollywood', while Arjun Kapoor 'responds with the jealous rage that heroes have traditionally exhibited for their female love interests'. The two even 'drink from one heart-shaped glass and sleep together in one bed, wearing matching pyjamas that have enormous hearts positioned right over their bums'. The big fight between the two characters has Ranveer Singh take off his shirt while Arjun Kapoor watches him and smiles:

> They stare at one another, take a deep breath and then charge at one another in such a way that one has a fistful of the other's shirt in his clutch. With a smooth flourish, they disentangle, leaving both men shirtless, their shiny, oily torsos glistening expectantly. All this is done in slow motion, naturally.

Controversial historical drama and blockbuster movie *Padmaavat* (2018) received a comparable analysis by writer Sandip Roy, who discussed the subversive aspects of the movie in an article for *Firstpost* as well. Roy argues: 'The film is so over-the-top, it veers into camp.' While the lead actress Deepika Padukone remains covered from head to toe, even in one of the movie's most iconic dancing scenes, 'the men are all heaving bare chests, always happy to soak in a bathtub or take a break from battle to wrestle glossily ... No bosom heaves as much in the film as the pectorals of Ranveer Singh and Shahid Kapoor as they go mano-a-mano, seemingly drawn to each other by some inexorable force of animal magnetism.' In fact, Roy notes, the two 'even go to great lengths to be alone together, their faces inches away from each other'. To Roy, the movie is 'the stuff of gay fantasies'.[210]

Faced with the jocular but insistent inquiries from gay friends, whose casual banter had followed me over the years as I looked into the emergence of a fitness and bodybuilding scene in India, I had to confront my own set of gay fantasies as well. As much as I had been all set to approach the topic on hand with the kind of clinical analytical gaze required by my profession, I also realised that, as an anthropologist, my own gaze mattered as well. Surely I found some of these men attractive, my Delhi friend once rather exasperatedly asked. Indeed, there was no point in denying that. However, encountering these men up-close at bodybuilding competitions, where they were covered in tanning lotion, their bodies strong yet weak, the penetrating smell of protein powder inescapable, and paper-thin skin revealing the ravaging effect of acne (usually the result of steroid use), had also shot holes in this gay fantasy.

As I hung out endlessly in gyms, I was never not aware that to be an openly gay researcher would make everything I wanted to know about the topic suspect. Once, a senior bodybuilder, who was about to advise a new disciple on which anabolic steroids and growth hormones to use, suddenly demanded to know if I was gay. He had been a friend on Facebook for a while, and even though he had thousands of such online friends, something must have triggered this question. I quickly confirmed that I was, but that this was not the reason why I had become interested in the topic, something he accepted without further ado. A somewhat warbled account of a bodybuilder who had been found to render same-sex services backstage at a competition somewhere in Tamil Nadu followed. It had 'deeply disgusted' him, not because he was against 'the gays', but because sex had no place at such an event to begin with. It was precisely what I had been so adamantly keeping out of my own analysis as well, realising full well that this was an often unspoken opinion across the bodybuilding and fitness spectrum. Yet, the very absence and presence of sexual desire and activities did inform the production of these muscular bodies so ubiquitously on display across urban India.

## HOMOEROTIC DESIRE AND HOMOSOCIAL BONDING

Within the gym, the talk about building bodies, about breaking the body down or even demolishing it, produces a lingo of construction that mingles and merges with the hammering and drilling of building sites in the background. Yet, these lean, muscular bodies are not merely a product of new India; they are also repositories of people's imaginations and fantasies that know a much longer history. The homoerotic layering of photographs and other depictions of muscle- or strongmen has long been a topic of fascination for historians and aficionados alike. In an insightful study titled *Universal Hunks* (2013), author David L. Chapman, who also published an influential biography on Eugen Sandow (1994), brings together the pictorial history (1895–1975) of muscular men from around the world. In the foreword, sports historian Douglas Brown raises the question of what a hunk actually is, pointing at the very subjectivity of hunkiness itself. While this might indeed be a matter of individual interpretation, the photographs selected are all of decidedly muscular men whose framing conveys a heady mix of admiration and adulation. Without explicitly stating this, the male gaze is circuitously present and there is an undercurrent of same-sex desire that seems to have profoundly influenced the curation of the book. Even the very word 'hunk' points to this—something a magazine such as *Men's Health* staunchly avoids, having always made it a point not to be seen as a 'gay magazine'.[211]

One set of photographs in *Universal Hunks* is of the Bangalorean bodybuilder K.V. Iyer (1897–1980), who featured occasionally in American and British muscle magazines in the 1930s. Iyer also wrote books on health and bodybuilding, and contributed to the Indian magazine *Vyayam* (Physical Training). Allegedly, he was well aware 'of his own beauty' and claimed that he had 'a body which gods covet'.[212] Most of the pictures included in *Universal Hunks* are not nudes. Almost all men don either posing slips, underwear or have their private parts covered with a leaf of some variety. Douglas Brown notes that '[E]ach photograph is inter-textual and, at any moment in time, is admired or scrutinized according to a multitude of shifting ideas about health and fitness, male beauty, masculinity, sexuality, pleasure, and desire'.[213] He warns that, like literary texts, they build on pre-existing codes, discourses and other texts. It is an observation that resonates with the analysis author Erick Alvarez provides in *Muscle Boys* (2008), with its focus on gay gym culture. Interviewing Robert Mainardi, author of *Strong Men: Vintage Photos of a Masculine Icon* (2001), Alvarez poses the question of whom these pictures were intended for. Mainardi explains that most were meant to be sold to women but that many also ended up in collections owned by men.

However, he hesitates labelling these men as gay per se, since the concept of homosexuality itself was poorly developed at the time.[214] That said, strongmen photography did pave the way for homoerotic media later on.[215] Until the 1920s, such photography contributed to the idea that one could appreciate a man for being handsome. However, with the arrival of Charles Atlas (1892–1972), an Italian-American bodybuilder born Angelo Siciliano, there was a gradual shift in thinking in terms of the way the muscular body speaks to or denies homosexuality. In the infamous marketing campaign, Charles Atlas contrasted scrawny, 'sissy' guys with far more successful muscular 'real' men, suggesting muscularity as an antidote or cure to manly underperformance.[216]

Bodybuilding continues to be characterised by an ambivalent relationship with same-sex desire and admiration, something already underlined in anthropologist Alan Klein's classic study *Little Big Men* (1993), which focused on the West Coast bodybuilding scene. While some of the bodybuilders in his study were involved in sex work, such as offering their bodies for 'muscle worship' to male clients, same-sex desire and homosexuality remained taboo topics in the gym. Gender scholar Ellexis Boyle (2010) points out that there is a homoerotic paradox or contradiction in bodybuilding that arises from the fetishisation of the male body as well as the intimate relationships that men develop in all-male sporting cultures.[217] Therefore, homosocial bonding and homoerotics often appear in a dialectic though not always amicable relationship with each other. If one contrasts this with the depictions of Greek gymnasiums and its sportsmen in its earliest days, one sees that this relationship has gradually become unhinged. Joseph Alter (2005) notes that Athenian gymnasiums were places where men came to become men and to develop themselves into citizens. Plato and Aristotle thought of gyms as institutions of embodied knowledge, something that has progressively been filtered out of modern philosophical thinking.[218] The depiction of naked wrestlers, often referred to as an early source of homoerotic contemplation and desire—with the penis clearly visible— needs to be understood within a context whereby the sexual relationship between older and younger men was understood as central to an embodied development of *arete*, or the idea of living up to one's full potential.[219] From this, it follows that we can understand the gym to be a place where men gave birth to men, as Alter also pointed out.

The gym as a space where men make men, give birth to them and themselves, finding their true selves that were hidden behind fat and weakness, is a train of thought that potentially stitches together a whole lot of assumptions about why men might be interested in building muscles. However, such reasoning often works better in theory than in practice. Theories such as those underpinning the idea of a crisis of masculinity[220] and the potential for homosocial bonding in gyms—away from the 'prying and judging eyes' of women and changing gender relations—works best when the gym is in fact a male-only space, which it rarely ever is, even in India. Besides, gyms in urban India are also meant to be safe spaces protected from the harsh gender relations outside. An important caveat, though, is that the one thing that is not left at the door is class difference itself. And this comes particularly to the fore when we look at the way same-sex desire operates inside as well as outside the gym with reference to the muscular bodies of lower-middle-class trainers and bodybuilders. Ambrish Bhatia's movies point to this, even if mainly employing a homophobic framework.

So how then do we understand the ostensibly 'straight' identities of trainers and bodybuilders in light of the occasionally explicitly homoerotic photoshoots they engage in? Explanations would generally and 'simply' hold that these men saw such photoshoots as an opportunity to showcase their bodily accomplishments, primarily via social media (Instagram, Facebook and more recently TikTok). Like bodybuilding competitions on stage, the suggestion that the audience's gaze could venture beyond mere physical appreciation was staunchly ignored and even rabidly dismissed as something that had either not occurred to them or something they were not interested in. In contrast, the sexually explicit comments that their social media posts generated confirmed that their audience often proceeded well beyond mere whistling. The rather explicit hashtags that bodybuilders themselves used in these posts, such as #sexybeast or #hotboy, also indicated a certain awareness of the sexualised or erotic qualities of their bodies. If the gym can be thought of as a space where men make men, these men are definitely engaged in producing men that cater to a diverse array of spectators, even if the presence of some of them is often only obliquely acknowledged.

## Understanding the Bodybuilder's Body

Research on bodybuilding has always been preoccupied with the question of gender and what the bodybuilder's body communicates. Media and film scholar Niall Richardson (2004), for one, argues that such a body can be considered a vehicle for the display of masculine power. At the same time, this notion is challenged by the bodybuilder's inherent passivity on stage, where it is objectified by those in attendance.[221] Central to any analysis of the bodybuilder's body is the way it deviates from the normal. It is a radically perplexing body that often triggers confusion and misperception among those who are not part of the sport themselves. As a gender-dissident body, it unites both feminine and masculine characteristics: curvaceousness, hairlessness and tanning lotions, combined with the harsh angular lines that characterise powerful muscles. In the gym, when a bodybuilder or trainer inspects himself—not rarely filmed by a workout partner, to be uploaded on social media—those present in the gym will find it hard to ignore this body. But is one supposed to look? And if one does, what is one supposed to see? What is being inspected and filmed is the progress made, a trajectory of transformation. However, the bodybuilder in question has no control over how the visual is consumed. The Indian wrestler's body presents a similar conundrum. It represents an older masculine ideal, one that never held the same middle-class appeal as the lean, muscular body does now. Yet, in its depictions as well as the way wrestlers relate to their bodies, we stumble upon a similar set of issues. In his insightful study of Indian wrestling, R. Sengupta wonders what sport is as vividly erotic as wrestling.[222] 'The tensions of wrestling's homoerotic power have rippled through the ages.' While the pehlwan's body continues to be a source of inspiration for amateur and professional photographers, often there is a disconnect between the homoerotic desire that such photography tends to ooze with—lusciously shot on the ghats of Varanasi or in rural akharas in Haryana—and the way Indian wrestlers relate to and engage with their own bodies.

James Alter's extensive body of work on the topic is particularly revealing here. Through an analysis of the history of jori club swinging[223] in akharas, Alter points at the way exercise itself can be understood as a way of man-making. Jori club swinging and/or the fashioning of the ideal-type male body through exercise can be thought of as a kind of symbolic onanism, where a man turns himself into a man.[224] Pehlwans live celibate lives and locate their strength in their semen, making retention integral to their life philosophy and the way they engage with their sport. Turning men into men by means of semen, Alter points at a sexual act that only matters at an abstracted symbolic level, whereby the sex and fluid substance in question is contained by the self. Control over the body and self are crucial here, something that characterises building muscular bodies as well.

Richardson (2004) notes that even if the bodybuilder's body radiates the illusion of phallic or masculine strength, his near-nakedness on stage invites what could be thought of as a castrating gaze, one that sees him in the nude, so to speak. In symbolic terms, this renders him sexually weak. While a bodybuilder disavows this gaze with the very flexing of his muscles, radiating strength and being the envy of those in the audience, the combination of judgement and the lack of control over what the audience may be admiring and desiring means that there is a certain tension built into the act of posing. Richardson argues that 'the very nature of a bodybuilding competition distresses the masculine paradigms of patriarchal society'.[225] The oblique heterocentrist representation in fitness and bodybuilding magazines can be understood as a way to deflect homoerotic connotations.

In his analysis, Richardson draws upon French psychoanalyst Jacques Lacan's conceptualisation of 'hysteria as gender confusion' in order to point at how we may understand the potential 'erotic numbness' that the audience might experience at a bodybuilding competition, unable to deal with the confusing interplay of masculine and feminine characteristics on display.[226] In my years of attending numerous bodybuilding competitions across India, I wasn't always able to equate this with the actual hysteria going on—crowds cheering loudly, whistling and hollering. This 'appreciation' from the audience informed the way bodybuilders, trainers and fitness enthusiasts 'performed' in photoshoots and presented themselves to a much larger online audience. The queer dimensions of muscular bodies seemed less about their potential to upset notions of masculinity and femininity, and much more about their appeal across a (de-)sexualised spectrum. Although they were often presented as sexually attractive, informants were not necessarily after 'sexual attraction' per se. Therefore, this sexual appeal was also not always interpreted as potential for 'actual sex'.

## Closeness and Intimacy as a Final Frontier

Inside the gym, though, ruminations of this kind would seem far more grotesque than the bodies on display. Even talking was often discouraged, considered a distraction from what the focus ought to be: whipping the body into shape and pushing its outer limits, at most pausing to reflect on the actual workout and to take a quick snapshot of the progress made for uploading online. In front of the mirror, the focus would be on the achievements so far and the muscle groups that still required 'work'. Conversations about physical dimensions and training routines could go on for hours, but what this masculine body was supposed to stand for was considered self-evident. As with the city itself, asking questions that attempted to penetrate the thick muscles and oiled skin just bounced or slithered off. It was as if to linger, pause and explore would reveal the queerness of it all. 'Obviously' this body was much stronger, more attractive and masculine than the weak and effeminate Indian body of the colonial past? It was 'definitely' to be preferred over the post-Independence middle-class potbelly that had once signalled health and prosperity. There was 'surely' no doubt that 'this' fast-moving new India was to be desired over a sluggish post-Liberalisation India, shackled by Licence Raj and bureaucratic incompetence? Adopting a queer gaze helps move away from the 'ostensiveness' that characterises this kind of reasoning. It takes the sheen of obviousness off all this, so to speak.

The question of sexuality and sexual attractiveness was generally considered a non-topic within gyms and at bodybuilding competitions. Whether in the gym or on stage, the body was to be examined, studied, analysed and dissected in purely physical terms. While sitting next to jury members, I found that their judgement often alternated between appreciation for a particularly 'massive chest' or 'awesome triceps' and far more dismissive remarks about 'skinny legs' or 'weird nipples' (the latter often a result of 'juicing'). But on social media, these same bodies drew a highly sexualised reaction. The comments sections had many in the overwhelmingly male audience judging them in terms of sexual attractiveness and potency. My 'straight' informants seemed unperturbed by this. A lack in fluency in the English language sometimes simply meant that the message had not come across. More often, however, was the very possibility of a sexual encounter itself deemed too far-fetched. The lack of time, and the need to invest money and energy in building the body, were also why they didn't have girlfriends, I was often told. It would just impede their work as trainers and/or progress as bodybuilders.

As always, there was another side to the story as well, a contradiction that would gradually emerge the more I probed. Rather dismissively, trainer Srivat once pointed at a number of muscular youngsters working out in his gym, saying that for them it was 'just about impressing the girls', something he as an accomplished bodybuilder frowned upon. Naturally, a difference in age played a role in this, not to mention the fact that he was married, had two young children and was faced with the financial burden of having recently opened his own gym. However, his next remark that 'it's about show-off' and that 'they want that body to boast' complicates matters. Within a context of limited possible contact between young men and women—certainly those of lower-middle-class 'vernacular' backgrounds—the very fact of being noticed adds to what could be understood as 'masculine worth' among young Indian men. While gender relations are gradually changing in urban India, as with other processes of change that touch the lives of individuals, this change does not necessarily keep pace with that of the transformation of urban space itself. It was within this context that 'getting noticed' mattered, something the casual glance of a girl who might notice one's pronounced biceps or powerful chest may confirm, but which required the confirmation that other men had noticed 'her glance' as well. As one young fitness enthusiast who regularly worked out in a gym in Santacruz (Mumbai) once formulated it, 'I like it when they see me [meaning girls], my friends all notice it.'

The awareness of a more sexualised gaze was only ever diffidently admitted to, and sexual encounters within the gym or between trainers and clients even less so. If at all, such accounts were rarely recounted in a boisterous or positive manner. The difference in social and economic standing between the two was a crucial factor, of course. Referring to a colleague, a twenty-five-year-old trainer in Delhi once mentioned that 'he is very good with the ladies, they all want him'. It turned out that he provided training at home on the side, which the trainer I interviewed somewhat cynically described as 'yoga', mimicking quotation marks with his fingers. But it was better that the gym they worked for should not find out. 'It is not encouraged, they warn us against it.'

A twenty-seven-year-old trainer working in a high-end gym in Gurgaon, explained that 'we are not to get too close to our clients'. Again, management was very particular about this. 'There have been some complaints,' he added. 'Some issue was there, but we should not be talking about this.' When I probed a little deeper, it turned out that there had been an affair between a married customer and her personal trainer. 'There had been complaint, that guy is no longer with us.' While the complaint had boiled down to harassment, according to the trainer his colleague had simply misinterpreted the one-night stand he had had with his client. 'He was very much in love with her, he would send her lots of messages.' She had clearly not appreciated this. While the informant who recounted this saga spoke of 'company policy' that prohibits such encounters between clients and employees, he nonetheless understood the negative outcome mainly in terms of class difference. When I mentioned the incident to a friend who regularly updated me about his own sexual encounters with lower-middle-class men across town, he laughed heartily and pointed out: 'Well, there you have the limitations of social mobility!' Indeed, it did seem to be a boundary not to be crossed. Closeness and intimacy across class boundaries could even be thought of as the final frontier here.

## Capitalising on Sexual Attractiveness

About a month after our initial conversation via Instagram and WhatsApp, I contacted Selvam to ask about his recent participation in a fitness event in Goa, which he quickly dismissed as 'ridiculous', suggesting it was more like a marketing event. Apparently, the focus had not been on the participants but the organisers and participating celebrities instead. 'We were just secondary. So typical Indian, in a way.' Over dinner with two other participants from Delhi, the conversation had turned to the topic of sex work. Selvam described how the conversation between the two trainer-models progressed: 'If someone from the organisation wanted to enjoy with them in exchange for some benefits, they were open to it,' he said. What made this particularly interesting to Selvam was that 'most of the participants were already known to some of the organisation'. His two dinner partners had, in fact, managed to claim first and third place in the category they participated in. 'So I cannot say directly, but yes, there is lots going on ... people in the fitness industry kind of assume that they need to do stuff.'

Once again, Selvam stressed that they do not see it as something gay; 'it's just the way it is'. He added that 'in fitness case, it's also the acknowledgement that people are ready to pay to enjoy your body'. Furthermore, he felt that 'money is a force more powerful than ethics ... Very few people have a profound incorruptible moral ground'. In fact, at the time, he was convinced that most fitness trainers are into 'it' one way or another, and that the balance between money vs name is an important consideration here. 'If you are sexy, you keep getting these offers from eager men. And if one day it hits you in a low financial moment, you just go for it.' In that sense, he really didn't 'know a single guy who hasn't done some kind of escorting at some point of time'. Yet, he also admitted that even he usually heard about this 'via 3rd parties', meaning that it did not concern first-hand accounts. 'It's kind of a shameful activity for many', since 'your manliness might be in question', as 'everybody knows that with a client you need to be flexible'. This entails doing 'some things you wouldn't do as a straight macho man', something that he also considers himself to be. 'It is performance', to which he adds: 'But as in every performance, sometimes might be more or less pleasant.'

A year later, we meet in the bar in Chennai as I mentioned earlier. By this time, it appears, he has been able to build himself a network of trainers who may be interested in generating an income as he does. His *Only Fans* account has been doing well, and 'others' have clearly taken inspiration from it, 'attempting the same'. He now collaborates with some of these trainers for sex scenes, to which he adds, 'If I like somebody, I can do very satisfying.' It remains unclear to what extent he feels alienated from his own sexual identity in this process. 'Gay for pay' though he is, Selvam doesn't necessarily appear to *not* enjoy it. Yet, when I inquire what he prefers, he breaks down. With tears in his eyes, he recounts how he got married when he was nineteen as part of a strategy to alleviate the family's burden of debts. 'She was my uncle's daughter and we had taken a loan with him.' That the loan was no longer a cause for concern could be thought of as dowry here. He has a young daughter now, and without further ado fishes out his cell-phone to show me a video of her dancing in his living room. Then he excuses himself to wash his face in the bathroom. When he returns, Selvam explains that this is very emotional for him, and that his wife does not know about the work he does. 'She is not aware of this at all, she does not know what that is.' He is very particular about keeping it that way, even if there is the constant danger that word might travel back to their native place on the outskirts of Chennai. That he uses his actual name as part of his social media presence and pornographic work does not make this any easier, something he knows too. At the same time, he also feels a certain pride in how he has persevered, thinking of himself as a survivor who has nothing to be ashamed of. He loves his wife, would rather wake up next to her every day, but is also taking care of his family in a way that his father never did. He feels it gives him 'some leverage' to make his own decision about how he actually does this. As he puts it succinctly: 'If they [meaning the larger family] have a problem with it, they will be begging on the streets.' But he was not particularly worried that they might find out about his erotic modelling and sex work: 'They are all villagers, so not much into social media, etc.' At the same time, he has no doubt that some of the photos will find their way to them at some point. It is an inevitability he has to prepare himself for. He feels, 'It's all about the balance between money and name (reputation).' He compares himself with middle-class folk whose financial situation is under less strain. 'When there are dire financial needs, Indians will be ready to do anything,' adding defiantly, 'and fuck the name, regrets may come later on, but that's how it is.'

## BRIDGING THE OSTENSIBLE GAP IN MIDDLE-CLASSNESS

While all three men discussed in this chapter capitalise on the sexual attractiveness of their bodies in one way or another, Selvam is the only one who has actually resorted to providing escort work, something the others vehemently deny ever having engaged in. Still, their homoerotically saturated photoshoots utilise sexual capital to further their ambition, whether it is to enlarge their personal training client base or source 'lucrative' modelling assignments. While Selvam was adamant about his belief that most trainers had at some point involved themselves in sex work-related activities, he also admitted that information about this had often reached him via third parties, meaning he did not know the person in question. Even if gay friends emphasised the easy availability of trainers for sexual services, I often found direct accounts and experiences lacking. I couldn't help think of it as an urban fantasy that was revealing for the way upper-middle-class men thought of lower-middle-class men whose bodies they admired and sexually desired, but whose position in society they certainly did not envy. In fact, for most of their lives, they had been used to these 'lower classes' catering to their every need: as drivers, cooks, gardeners, security guards, tutors and so on.

Instead of focusing on the 'truth' here, the question of the availability of fitness trainers and bodybuilders for sex work should be considered in light of the puzzle of a changing India itself. As this book has argued throughout, India's change does not necessarily translate to the same pace at an individual level, where things move slowly. The way new middle-class professionals, such as Selvam, Bikram and Girish, make use of the opportunities that a new India presents them with is not generalisable per se.

Selvam's sister's suicide profoundly impacted the family and made an already precarious financial situation worse. His marriage at nineteen only partly solved their predicament, and Selvam feels the weight of his family's obligations on his muscular shoulders every day.

Bikram's father passed away and left his mother and siblings in a financially precarious situation. He knows that whatever financial risk he takes next—venturing into sportswear or building a fitness brand for himself—will impact those he has vowed to take care of.

Girish's ambitions to become a competitive bodybuilder requires a considerably higher financial investment than what Bikram and Selvam need to maintain their muscular bodies. His limited personal training client-base cannot nearly provide for this, and as a result, he remains dependent on his family when a 'man his age' should be starting a family of his own. Besides financial constraints, his usage of anabolic steroids and growth hormones might render this impossible in the longer term as well.

All three, however, now make considerably more per month than their parents ever did, and are able to afford lifestyles that were previously unheard of in their families and communities. In their attempts at upward mobility in a 'new India', these accounts continue to tell of the roadblocks and boundaries to be negotiated along the way. While they are part of a muscular India, flexing admirably large muscles that are desired at multiple levels, this same India with its inherent class hierarchies does not hesitate to flex its own muscles as well. India is never not its own muscular doorman that way.

Having read one of my earlier publications, Selvam once messaged that, even though he didn't reach twelfth standard, 'I guess I am just an extreme case of what you so inspiringly call "bridging the ostensible gap in middle-classness", to which he adds a '☺'. In this article I had argued that an 'ideal type' body alone was not enough to be successful in the Indian fitness industry. 'Equally if not more important was the way a trainer was successfully able to bridge the ostensible gap in middle-classness.'[227] It resonated with Selvam's own experiences, though in his ambition to make money and live the lifestyle of his 'clients', staying in high-end hotel rooms and traveling to lush locations across India, he had gone decidedly further than most others I met over the years. It had rendered him proud but also deeply cynical. At some point, during our long conversations about his work providing sexual services to male clients and uploading regular pornographic content to his *Only Fans* account, he said: 'We are tissue papers for clients to blow their noses in and then toss away.' While it is probably unnecessary for me to explain what exactly he meant by 'blowing their noses' here, it did point at something that resonated through other accounts of fitness trainers as well: that as unique as their bodies may be, they were also ultimately replaceable.

# EPILOGUE

In 2018, I take a taxi from Bangalore airport to the suburb of RT Nagar to visit my in-laws. The urban landscape has changed dramatically once again. However, this time it is not the ongoing urban sprawl that catches my attention. Normally, the city greets visitors first with towering billboards advertising a whole array of goods and services, but this time they are all gone. Threads of former advertisements dangle haphazardly in the wind, giving Bangalore the feel of an abandoned frontier ghost town.

A Google search reveals that a ban had been issued on commercial hoarding within the Bruhat Bengaluru Mahanagara Palike (BBMP) area, excluding areas such as MG Road and Brigade Road. Gone are the advertisements for the construction of new apartment complexes with fancy European-sounding names; the announcements for new McDonald's and KFC menus have disappeared; and the sculpted men advertising a whole gamut of products from deodorant to holidays in Goa and Kerala are gone. Like the construction projects, cars on the road, and Café Coffee Days flanking the roads, these billboards had always appeared to have multiplied each time I visited the city.

As much as I wondered about these ghostly billboards, my family and friends in the city took little notice. It was mainly perceived as a glitch, a short interruption of business as usual. Surely, this was some political stunt, somebody trying to make money, I was assured. These billboards would be up in no time. This was not something that would last. Just wait and see!

The idea of a new India almost automatically evokes the notion of speed—things happening in a hurry, faster than they can be tracked. It appears that research somehow needs to mirror that speed. How else can we understand what's going on? This book shows that the speed of change at an individual level rarely meets the speed with which things appear to be changing in general. There is an important reason for using 'appear' here because the narrative of a changing or new India is one that could do with a healthy dose of nuance. Sure, India is in motion, but wasn't it always? Late professor Mario Rutten, an expert on Gujarat and a dear friend, once remarked that it had always struck him as fundamentally flawed to argue that 'things were really changing now' in India. They had always been changing, he felt, nothing had ever been set in stone, there had never not been a time when everything was heading in a completely different direction from before. It was something he had observed over decades of spending significant amounts of time in second-tier towns such as Anand and elsewhere in semi-rural Gujarat. This doesn't mean, of course, that change is not real, and that people don't need to find a way to deal with the changes they face in their lifetimes.

That is why, I will wind up this tale with an impression of how the lives of the men discussed in *Muscular India* have developed since we met them last. These men's trajectories are principally ongoing, of course. Like arriving at a comprehensive estimate of the size of the Indian middle class, an answer to the questions I have raised throughout the book will never quite be able to capture the complexity of a society in motion, of how illusive yet massive, how slippery and truly momentous change is.

## The 'Classic' Aspirations of Akash

Following my encounter with empty billboards, I meet Akash for lunch at the same place in Indiranagar we had gone to earlier. As he walked in earlier than expected, I couldn't help noticing how he looked even bigger than before. Truly enormous arms, colossal biceps and a gigantic chest, he clocked 112 kg at the time, even though the competition-category he was aiming for was in the 90 kg range. It was not something he was particularly worried about, he explained. During this bulking phase, he was enjoying not having to worry about every bite that went into his mouth and was keen to devour one of the restaurant's famous burgers.

The previous year, Akash had competed in his first international competition, held in Mongolia. By the time he reached Ulan Bator, he realised he would have to lose another 10 kg if he were to have any chance of reaching the top three at all. He eventually managed to pull it off with the help of diuretics and steam baths. 'I was being cooked man, I was in that steam bath the whole time!' But it was also during the Mongolia competition that he started to realise that he was not nearly big enough yet. In his own weight class of 90-plus kg, there were 'much bigger guys, much more muscular!' He did enjoy competing because the atmosphere was so different from that of India, where he had found his fellow competitors to be 'nasty and aggressive'. Yet something had changed in terms of what he saw himself aiming for in the coming years.

In Mongolia, he had learned of the so-called Arnold Classic category for the first time. He described it as 'going back to the figures and posing of the 1980s, basically what Schwarzenegger looked like'. It is something he now wants to achieve for himself as well. 'When you are this big, nothing is easy, you know.' When he had lost weight for the competition, he noticed how much easier certain things were, even if he felt completely depleted of any energy. 'Now I am putting all this weight on me, my knees are taking a beating as well.' But he also appreciates the aesthetics of it more. 'It is not just about becoming huge, it just looks better.' He pulled out his phone to illustrate what he meant.

After the two competitions he still has lined up, Akash is contemplating becoming smaller, not bigger. He has discussed this with his Australian coach to whom he pays Rs 10,000 per month for online advice. He hoped to derive an income out of a similar scheme himself someday, saying: '... he doesn't need to work all that much for it.' Turning to a 'more natural look' and participating in Arnold Classic-like competitions would also help his online appeal internationally, he felt.

Even though he was still employed by the same Gold's Gym, the idea of starting his own fitness business had become more concrete. An additional reason for this was the politics and favouritism he had encountered at the gym, which was beginning to get to him. He still wasn't meeting his targets, but he had been consistent with his results, so his clients liked coming back to him. He was now a Super Platinum category trainer, above which there is only one more category. But he was not sure if he wanted to 'take' that category because it was very hard to get people to pay so much for training. 'Only really rich people can afford that.' It comes down to about Rs 70,000 for twelve sessions. It still amazes Akash that new trainers hardly seem to possess any real knowledge of how bodies function and transform, in spite of the certificates they boast of.

Akash feels he has the body to show for his knowledge. However, he also realises that others may think his physique was built only on juice. The idea amuses him and strikes him as ridiculous. 'They have no idea how many hours we put in the gym to get there. How much time, energy ... how much we give up for it.' Coming to the topic of the risks bodybuilders take, the conversation turns to a bodybuilder from Mumbai who had supposedly used synthol to make his muscles look bigger. 'So many are dying now.' It was something he kept hearing about all the time, and which had made him even more determined to— eventually—focus on a 'healthier' massively muscular body.

## RIP Samson Solomon

My very first informant and dear friend Samson Solomon (real name) passed away early September 2018. Like so many, I had first met Samson on Facebook where he posted regular updates of his progress as an aspiring bodybuilder. The first time we met, he drove me around on his motorcycle, which barely supported his colossal physique, and showed me his old bodybuilding haunts in Mumbai. Through him, I came to know an older generation of bodybuilders and fitness enthusiasts who provided a glimpse into the sport's much longer history in India. In those early days, Samson was not particularly successful in deriving an income as a fitness and personal trainer. He often complained that high-end chains like Gold's Gym were not interested in his services because they were afraid that his enormous body might scare off customers. 'They don't like to be associated with that,' he suggested, adding: 'They think I am a monster.'

When I went to Delhi to start my fellowship with Nalanda University in 2013, Samson had just moved there himself, and was now living close to his best friend, female bodybuilder Rita Singh. He shared his house with four enormous dogs and twenty birds, including cockatoos and macaws. Even if he was involved in various fitness-related businesses, his own bodybuilding career was faltering. He had started injecting synthol to enlarge his muscles, which made them look odd and ill-proportioned. As a result, he was frequently denied entry into competitions, something that weighed heavily on him.

Samson died while sedated during a routine treatment to deal with a deviated septum, which he had had since childhood. The bodybuilding community was quick to link his synthol-use to his untimely passing, even if it appeared not to have been a factor in his death. It did, however, underline how the sport continues to struggle with health-related issues and how the pursuit of bigness is rarely just about the man in the mirror, but also the reflection of oneself in the eyes of one's community.

## VICTOR CONTINUES HIS WAY UP

When I met Victor in 2018, he had just learned of Samson Solomon's death and was keen to share his opinion with me. Well aware of synthol use among aspiring bodybuilders, his critique was not so much about its use but the way people professed to know the way it operated in the body. He had recently taken over the branding and activities of a well-known gym chain in Chennai, and continued to combine this with providing personal training on the side. His income was much higher by this time than it had ever been when he was working for PayPal, and his family no longer doubted that he had made the right decision.

But his relationship with various bodybuilding federations and associations remained acrimonious. He experienced considerable backlash from 'the old guard' when he recently organised a competition without their backing. In fact, he even received some thinly veiled threats on social media to underline their dismay. However, he remains committed to freeing the sport from the 'corrupt' involvement of those who only care to see their own people win, as he puts it.

Now that he is also involved in the training of talent outside the field of fitness and bodybuilding, who may eventually qualify for the Summer Olympics in Tokyo, he is branching out in a way few of his competitors have. His Instagram account now counts over half a million followers. Key to building this following have been regular videos, in which he provides diet advice, workouts and other health-related matters. His own incredibly muscular physique fuels 'his brand' as much as it raises questions about how much longer he will be able to maintain it in its current form.

## Raj Shining on Stage

Raj did shine on stage eventually—not once but several times. A picture he sent me at some point shows him posing victoriously backstage. He had indeed put on considerable mass and it looked like his decision to invest in growth hormones had paid off. More recently, he informed me of his decision to move away from bodybuilding and to focus on his IT career full-time. Even if he continued to attend the same gym and train under Srivat, his new position in handling automation and robotics was demanding his undivided attention.

When I met him for lunch in 2018, he cheerfully commented that I had put on weight since he last saw me, even if his own weight-gain was not particularly easy to ignore either. As a researcher, surely I had plenty of time to keep myself fit, he reasoned. He himself was faced with the busy demands of his job and the challenge of keeping a regular schedule with the gym. It is a predicament that continues to dominate our conversations on WhatsApp, even if I am unlikely to ever come close to the figure he once sported. I sometimes remind him of the question he once asked me, about what I would do if I had his body. I distinctly remember telling him that I would have signed up a long time ago, but the kind of discipline and dedication he had put into building his muscles was something that would never come 'natural' to me. Even if his bodybuilding career had not been particularly 'natural' either, what he had accomplished was self-evident. The occasional glances from co-workers confirmed that he hadn't completely lost what he had so carefully built over all these years.

## Manish in Search of the Next Opportunity

In 2019, I caught up with Manish in Delhi. He had just taken over general management of a new gym in Gurgaon; a highly specialised, high-end one that makes use of Spanish technology imported from Dubai. While visiting Manish at his new gym, I also met the investor in the project, part of a Dubai-based business family that was originally from Delhi. He immediately started probing me about whether I could help him with any leads into the 'Singapore market', which he considered very promising. I was quickly given the run down and sales pitch, during which I watched Manish's usual confidence and patience diminish.

When his investor left for an 'urgent' appointment, I asked Manish why he did not seem his usual self. 'That guy is all about business, no emotions,' he answered. I had always known Manish to be a salesperson himself, but over lunch at a burrito place nearby, he explained that he had serious reservations about the project. Earlier he had asked me to participate in a trial of an odd-looking suit with electrodes attached to various body parts. An incredibly sweaty contraption to be in, the idea was that the suit would give small electric shocks to the different muscle groups while working out. It would make weight loss and building muscles much easier while it was also supposed to prevent potential injury. It seemed an incredibly complex and invasive way to work on one's health, and I wondered who would be willing to go through the hassle of putting on the suit every time and pay the rather exorbitant fees—something Manish did not seem entirely convinced about either.

Evidently, he was still searching for an alternative after his involvement with BodyHolics came to an end. As usual the conversation turned to 'the gym', and how he missed his trainers and clients. His emotions also got the better of him when he stated that he 'helped everybody but when I needed help nobody helped me'. It had hugely disappointed him. Long-term members had complained that he had taken their membership fees in advance, and that when the gym closed, he had not been able to return this money. He had hoped for their understanding, but it had tarnished his name instead.

Before taking up management of this high-tech gym in Gurgaon, he had managed a gym called Chisel, which was started by Virat Kohli. When we drove down to a nearby market, he pointed at the gym, which was located on top of a branch of 24/7 Fitness. Again, it struck me how fitness chains themselves had increased over the years. Near BodyHolics, two new gyms had established their businesses. Manish still does not like driving down that road because of the emotions it brings back.

Recently, he consulted a numerologist and concluded that he is 'a very emotional guy' who sees enemies everywhere, even though he is a hard worker.

I couldn't but help notice how Manish looked strangely tired. His sister had recently got married and, as usual, the family had knocked on his door for money because of his image as a money-maker. 'There is always something that needs taken care of,' he said and sighed. But he felt very proud and content that his sister was now married because 'that was a huge responsibility for me'. The family still resides in Chirag Dilli, a hundred metres from Amit, with whom he is still in touch. They had briefly collaborated to provide personal training to the CEO of Amazon India. 'I learnt so much from that guy!' Contemplating this some more, he added: 'Most people will beg to get five minutes with him, but I was able to establish a real relationship. When you talk to him, he will explain things with hundred things connected. He is like that.' Meanwhile, Manish was exploring various alternative business options, having little faith that the current gym he was managing would take off. Indeed, it wasn't long before he started another business, this time in event management, with which he hoped to venture well beyond the confines of 'just' fitness and bodybuilding.

## Amit as a Poor Man with Three Cars

I had met Amit at various intervals earlier and he would usually invite me to his home in Chirag Dilli. The first time I had to find my way there, I got completely lost in the narrow alleyways and eventually had to text him my location on Google Maps so that he could come and find me. Unlike Manish, he had fully moved on from BodyHolics and rarely reflected on his time there. Whenever we met, he would briefly inquire if I was still in touch with some of the gym's regular clients, such as Supriya, who had since moved to Canada with her family.

Amit's personal training business had taken off, and it was something he combined with an involvement with the local chapter of the BJP. An avid supporter of India's prime minister, Narendra Modi, he had become involved in 'arranging' solutions for neighbours and community members whose financial situation might not be as flourishing as his own. For instance, if a family is short on dowry money, he operates a funding organisation that may be able to provide the couple with, say, a refrigerator. 'Or we give them some contribution to the wedding, like pay for the venue or dinner.'

Occasionally I see him post updates where his smiling face is plastered on some billboard next to a range of other local figures, adorned by a decidedly larger image of the prime minister himself. When I once remarked that he seemed to be doing well, Amit assured me that he was still a poor man— something I continue to tease him about because of what followed next. After having lunch at his family home, he offered to drive me to my next appointment at nearby Select Citywalk. When we walked down to a parking area nearby, he could not quite decide which car to use. There were three nearly identical Tata Indica's parked in a row, but the key he had brought along was only for one of them. The cars belonged to his family, he explained somewhat apologetically. He could use any one of them anytime. 'A poor man with three cars, huh?'

## SHIVAM IN THE NATIONAL CAPITAL REGION

Shivam was invariably enthusiastic every time I said I was coming to Delhi, promising me a wild night out or at least lunch at his place. It never quite happened as planned, which is something I had come to expect. Shivam's life was always in motion and there was never not a next 'big thing' waiting to happen. Most recently, we met in a mall in Gurgaon. He was there to discuss involvement in the business of air purifiers and water alkalisers. Though it was a deviation from his plans to set up a bodybuilding federation and organise fitness events, these plans had been far from shelved. When he gave me a bearhug as soon as I walked in, I felt the raw power in his biceps. It appeared he had returned to working out regularly. He launched immediately into his disappointment about having had to delay his plans. 'Indians are shit, man, I will tell you that.' They just didn't seem to understand his vision. 'One day I am going to be so big, you won't even believe it!' Arnold Schwarzenegger had done the same. He had gone from bodybuilding to Hollywood and then became a governor! Shivam imagined a similar trajectory for himself one day. Meanwhile, I learnt that Rajender Bainsla had taken up a political position—the responsibility for the maintenance of an upper-middle-class neighbourhood in South Delhi, not too far from where I had lived myself at some point. Cynically, Shivam put it as follows: 'So that's how it works: get some bodybuilders around you, build that network, and then say I can do this and this.' And that's what Bainsla had done, he said.

## KISHORE'S HAPPINESS FUCKED UP

I continue to see Kishore on regular visits to Mumbai, usually in Chembur, where he now runs a new gym. The last time I visited him, he had handed over day-to-day management to twenty-six-year-old Shalini, who grew up five minutes from his house in Chembur. Even if they had only known each other for three months, they appeared to be close business partners and avowed to have 'incredible faith' in each other. Shalini also knew Kishore's wife well and often ate at their place, even if his father apparently 'hated her' and often gave her a disapproving look.

I met her for the first time in 2018, arriving in Chembur from Bandra West. The Uber driver had considerable difficulty locating Kishore's new, semi-outdoor gym. Eventually 'things' had not worked out with the person who owned the wedding ground that he had previously used as a site, and this new place offered a more permanent home for his business.

Meanwhile, Shalini had tried calling me a few times already via WhatsApp to inquire where I was. It was a Sunday afternoon, and since the gym would close at three that day, she was worried I might not get to see the place in action. While we waited for Kishore to arrive, Shalini filled me in on her involvement in Kishore's gym. After seven years 'in media', and having worked with almost all of the Bollywood stars, she had felt it was time for a change. She grew up in Chembur, but unlike Kishore, she had attended an English-medium convent school; she clearly belonged to a different layer of middle-class society altogether. Her father is an important property developer in Chembur. Eager to convince me how close she had become with Kishore in a short period of time, even if he is clearly not of her world, she mentioned that they had hit it off almost immediately after she had joined his gym to lose weight. She no longer had the body for it, but she had been a Kingfisher calendar girl at some point, and was eager to get back in shape.

With the gym closed for the day, we decided to take an auto to a nearby bar that specialised in various types of craft beer. It was a place I had not imagined existed in Chembur, recalling the area's rather dingy 'old school' bars we usually frequented. The walls of this bar were adorned with advertisements for new types of brews, and it even seemed to work with a fancy system of bidding to determine the popularity and price of each beer.

Shalini appeared to frequent it quite regularly, but Kishore noticed my surprise to find him hanging out in a place like this. Growing up in a Rajput family, Shalini had dated a 'Marwari boy', but the relationship came to an untimely end when her mother made it clear that the family would never allow them to get married. Now in her late twenties, she felt she had lost considerable time on the wedding market. It was not hard to see how enthralled she had become with Kishore, pinching his biceps and eager to tell me how intimate she had become with his family. When I joked that she was like his second wife, both laughed loudly though, with an embarrassed smile, Kishore assured me nothing was going on. Over the course of the evening, however, it became clear that Kishore was not entirely convinced by what this alliance meant to him.

After having ordered our third round, Shalini started rolling up Kishore's T-shirt sleeves so that his biceps showed more clearly. She felt that he should show off more, even if I had never known Kishore to miss an opportunity to do so. His Facebook and Instagram accounts are still filled with almost daily updates of his body and athletic prowess. Apparently, she was keen on him participating in a Mr India competition, perhaps even progressing to Mr Olympia level. This puzzled me considerably since I knew he had always been quite concerned about steroid and hormone use. He was proud of his natural body, and bodybuilding had never been an ambition as far as I knew.

While she laid out her plans for him, I noticed him waiting for me to interrupt her lengthy explanation to ask the very obvious question about where all of this actually came from. When it came to steroids, he confessed that he was 'considering it' but that he was keen 'to maintain the youth' and not to 'become big'. It was clearly more her idea than his, and while she kept talking about this, he actually did not participate much in the conversation and looked unhappy.

There was a competition coming up in the next few months and she seemed to think that Kishore had a chance. At some point she said, 'I will fuck up his happiness in the next six months,' suggesting that she was really going to push Kishore to work harder on his body and to become more competitive. Throughout the evening, she referred to a recent event they had organised, and for which they had invited bodybuilder Rajesh Yadav. She had been quite impressed by the show he had delivered, and seemed to believe that Kishore could become 'like this' as well.

When I wondered out loud how he felt about the amount of 'juicing' required for this, Kishore confirmed that he had indeed always been uncomfortable about it. 'I have always been this guy, as long as Michael has known me, I have been like this.' His pride was centred on being able to maintain his body and the look of a fit and healthy guy, he said. He was well-aware that other men looked up to him for this. 'I have never been too keen to get so much into this medical stuff.'

The evening provided a snapshot from Kishore's ongoing journey, where he must negotiate questions of his body in relation to the path of upward socioeconomic mobility that he has been on for more than a decade. The 'relationship' with Shalini did not last long, and when I messaged both a few months later, it turned out she had left the gym to focus on 'other things', and Kishore was keen to forget about her involvement in his life altogether.

Shalini was clearly fascinated by Kishore's working-class background as well as his body, which she openly admired. I never quite understood what compelled her to give up her career in media to involve herself in the business of fitness, which she had no experience in, nor the body that one would expect for it. For Kishore, the deal was more clear-cut. Shalini's father was a leading property developer in Chembur, and a possible alliance with the family could help him sort out the nagging concern of the temporary nature that (again) characterised the place he rented at the time. Moreover, I knew he had plans to grow beyond just the one gym. Time will tell how he closes the gap in middle-classness that the brief involvement of Shalini once again accentuated.

## SELVAM IN CHAINS AND SHACKLED

In a particularly striking update on Instagram sometime in 2019, Selvam wears an elaborate gold chain around his waist; it almost looks like some sort of dowry contribution. Barely concealing his cock, it's a strikingly erotic picture that shows off his talent for taking incredibly suggestive pictures. In his right hand he holds a sword with the tip facing down, as if it were a walking stick. The picture is captioned: 'Warrior ready for battle.'

When I asked him for an update about his life by means of WhatsApp, he described it as 'OK, so I keep doing bold shoots'. He added that 'escort work has been a bit slow during summer'. The reason for this was that potential clients had gone off on holidays. 'But it's catching up again.' I was reminded of our discussion earlier, when he mentioned that it wouldn't surprise him if news of his activities found their way back to his native village.

'It did actually happen,' he responded almost immediately. 'It's unbelievable but it did.' Somehow, his pictures 'got into the hands of some gay fellows there'. And they had gone straight to his aunty. 'But I was able to manage.' She had clearly been scandalised, 'but then I explained that I was making money out of it'. As we discussed earlier, 'the money argument kinda softens everything up'. According to Selvam, poor people like his family understand this. 'Money talks and everything can be done for money ... And eventually money is stronger than morality.' The family is now aware of his 'modelling' activities, but not of the services he delivers as a sex worker. This is likely to change though since police officers have recently come to his door asking about his online activities, having been tipped off by what Selvam assumed to be a jealous cousin.

Rumours about sex work and the availability ('interest' in) same-sex contact continue to imbue the narrative and mythology that surrounds fitness trainers and bodybuilders in India. Even if Selvam emphasises that he knows of plenty of examples of men who are engaged in similar escort and 'modelling' work, most of this also reaches him via third parties. What it points to most of all is that, within the fast-changing context of a 'new India', there is little that is certain. Earlier, I drew the conclusion that these stories of the availability of trainers and bodybuilders for 'sexual services' signals an enduring, resilient internal hierarchy of what it means to be and belong to the middle class. The story of urban India and its associated fast-moving change is never completely told and finished.

# NOTES

1. It is furthermore suggested that the movie was inspired by the 1951 British movie *Happy Go Lovely,* which confusingly was itself loosely based on a German comedy from 1933 titled *And Who Is Kissing Me?.*
2. T.B. Macaulay's 'minute' is available at http://www.columbia. edu/itc/mealac/pritchett/00generallinks/macaulay/txt_ minute_education_1835.html (visited 24-10-2018).
3. Joshi, 2011: 83.
4. Ibid: 85.
5. Ibid: 2.
6. Varma, 1999: 157.
7. Gupta borrows the term westoxification from the Iranian intellectual Jala-e-Ahmed, referring to the so-called middle-class obsession with electronic goods, foreign brands and other aspects of 'modernity'. Also discussed in Belliappa, 2013: 10.
8. Mawdsley, 2004: 85, see also Mario Rutten, 2001.
9. P.R. Ramesh, 'Out to Bait the Middle Class', *Open,* 3 February 2014.
10. Ibid: 14. The drawing described is by Anirban Ghosh.
11. Ibid: 16.
12. See for a detailed analysis of the construction and layering of Brand Modi: *Business Today,* 'Just the Right Image', by Shamni Pande, available online: https://www.businesstoday.

in/magazine/case-study/case-study-strategy-tactics-behind-creation-of-brand-narendra-modi/story/206321.html (visited 11-02-2019).

13. *The Washington Post*, 'Modi Promises "Shining India" in Victory Speech', by Annie Gowen and Rama Lakshmi, available online: https://www.washingtonpost.com/world/hindu-nationalist-narendra-modis-party-heads-to-victory-in-indian-polls/2014/05/16/c6eccaea-4b20-46db-8ca9- af4ddb286ce7_story.html?noredirect=on&utm_term=.38fb63778d79 (visited 11-02-2019).

14. Shurmer-Smith, 2000: 29.

15. V.G. Kulkarni, 1993, 'The Middle Class Bulge', *Far Eastern Economic Review*, 156: 44.

16. Sheth, 1999: 337–333.

17. Fernandes, 2006: xiv.

18. Baviskar and Ray, 2011: 2.

19. E. Sridharan (2004). 'The Growth and Sectoral Composition of India's Middle Classes: Its Impact on the Politics of Liberalization in India', *India Review*, 3(4): 405–28; reprinted in *Elite and Everyman: The Cultural Politics of the Indian Middle Classes* (2011), edited by Amita Baviskar and Raka Ray, as 'The Growth and Sectoral Composition of India's Middle Classes: Their Impact on the Politics of Economic Liberalization', 27–57.

20. Dickey, 2012: 567.

21. Here Dickey refers to studies by Achin Vanaik, 'Consumerism and New Classes in India', in Sujata Patel, Jasodhara Bagchi, and Krishna Raj, eds, *Thinking Social Science in India: Essays in Honour of Allice Thorner* (New Delhi: Sage, 2002), 228; Satish Deshpande, *Contemporary India*, 2003: 134; William Mazzarella, *Shovelling Smoke: Advertising and Globalization in Contemporary India* (Durham, North Carolina: Duke University Press, 2003), 264–265. It thus needs to be noted that the studies that buttress the suggestion that the exaggeration of the higher numbers build on data that was gathered in the early 2000s.

22. Surinder S. Jodhka and Aseem Prakash, 2016: 7.

23. See Fernandes, Donner & De Neve, 2011: 4, referring to Appadurai, A. and Breckenbridge, C., 1995. 'Public Modernity in India', In: C. Breckenbridge (ed.) *Consuming Modernity: Public Culture in a South Asian World*. Minneapolis: University of Minnesota Press.

24. See Michiel Baas & Julien Cayla, 'Recognition in India's New Service Professions: Gym Trainers and Coffee Baristas', *Consumption Markets & Culture*, 2019, DOI: 10.1080/10253866.2019.1586678.

25. See for a more extensive discussion, Shurmer-Smith, 2000.

26. See among others Vinay Sitapati's (2016) *Half Lion: How P.V. Narasimha Rao Transformed India* (New Delhi: Penguin) and Jairam Ramesh's (2015) *To the Brink and Back: India's 1991 Story* (New Delhi: Rupa Publications).

27. All names in this book have been anonymised unless it concerned people whose reputation and ideas are commonly known and shared. Sometimes other aspects of informants' lives are changed as well to make sure their privacy is properly protected.

28. CR stands for Chittaranjan, while GK for Greater Kailash, the latter which consists of two parts. It is uncommon to refer to them by their full name.

29. As one of many urban villages in Delhi, Chirag Dilli was granted a special status as part of a city planning dilemma which revolved around how to categorise the various miscellaneous village settlements within the ever-expanding city.

30. See for a more detailed exploration of the symbolic value of the English language in India Chaise LaDousa's book *Hindi is Our Ground, English is Our Sky: Education, Language, and Social Class in Contemporary India* (New York: Berghahn Books, 2014); as well as Sazana Jayadeva's work on the topic (2018).

31. There are various spellings, such as gujar, gurjar, gurjjar, gojar, etc. Gujjar seems to be the most commonplace though.

32. All three are Tata brands.
33. Spaaij, 2011: 18. The field of cultural mobility studies is decidedly less 'systematically' developed.
34. See also Friedman, 2014: 356.
35. See also Bourdieu, 1993: 32–33.
36. Coleman, 1998, also discussed in Spaaij, 2011: 26-7.
37. Bourdieu, 1986, as also discussed in Spaaij, 2011: 25.
38. Episode 8, around 23:54.
39. Bourdieu, 1990: 56.
40. Thompson, 1991: 13.
41. Ganesh Chaturthi is the annually held ten- or eleven-day festival in celebration of the elephant god Ganesha. Though it is celebrated across India in a variety of ways, for Mumbai and Pune it is the most important festival of the year.
42. A murti is a general term for an image, statue or idol of a deity or mortal in Hinduism.
43. In Hinduism, a pandal is a temporary structure set up to venerate a deity.
44. During dry days, no liquor may be sold in shops, restaurants or bars.
45. The diversity in terms of customs during the festival is partly the product of the history of Ganesh Chaturthi itself and the way it evolved over time as a city-wide practice. See among others here a recent article in the *Hindustan Times* titled 'How Ganesh Chaturthi celebrations have evolved over time', to be found here: https://www.hindustantimes.com/mumbai-news/history-of-ganesh-chaturthi-from-uniting-indians-to-helping-parties-reach-out-to-masses/story-IeVHulDmbUJfv3iQyYgTrN.html (visited 08-03-2018).
46. Kollywood, the Tamil movie industry, is named after the suburb of Kodambakkam in Chennai where most of the industry is located.
47. The Indian edition of *Men's Health* ceased publication in September 2015.

48. Instead of thinking of globalising forces as principally homogenising, from the 1990s studies have increasingly described the way such globalisation 'lands' locally in terms of heterogeneity, meaning that the specific form it takes locally differs from location to location.

49. An article in *The Guardian* titled 'Brawn again: why Hollywood's muscle heroes are bigger than ever' (18-09-2018) notes that we are (again) in the 'age of the strongman'. It referenced Mark Wahlberg's daily fitness and dietary regime which includes two gym sessions, six meals and one hour cultivating his chest making use of a cryogenic recovery chamber. The author Alex Hess argues that 'a man's cultural worth these days can be accurately gauged by the circumference of his biceps.' Yet it must be noted that all the actors the article lists, ranging from The Rock to Van Diesel, are known for their roles as action heroes.

50. See for instance 'Farhan Akhtar is more ripped in "Wazir" than he was in "Bhaag Milkha Bhaag" says his fitness trainer Samir Jaura', http://www.thehealthsite.com/news/farhan-akhthar-fitness-wazir-bhaag-milkha-bhaag-samir-jaura-k1214/(visited 14-06-2017).

51. See for instance 'Celebrity diet and fitness secrets by Samir Jaura', http://timesofindia.indiatimes.com/life-style/health-fitness/fitness/Celebrity-diet-and-fitness-secrets-by-Samir-Jaura/articleshow/48342773.cms (visited 14-06-2017).

52. The first was published by Simon & Schuster, the latter by Om Books International.

53. 'Automatic Bodies' by Paromita Vohra, *The Indian Quarterly*, available online: http://indianquarterly.com/automatic-bodies/ (visited 26-03-2019). It's interesting to compare this to how Mukul Kesavan discusses the issue in *The Ugliness of the Indian Male and Other Propositions* (2008): '... with a few exceptions (Dilip Kumar was a persuasively broody lover, Dharmendra was an old-fashioned hunk, Shashi Kapoor was the pretty boy

par excellence, and Aamir and Shahrukh have some claim to cuteness) the men who figure in it [Bollywood] are, by most standards of male beauty, aggressively unbeautiful. Ashok Kumar was a charming man, but he had the physical presence of a cupboard wearing a dressing gown. Kundan Lal Saigal was possibly the ugliest leading man in the history of world cinema. Rajesh Khanna, the first superstar, looked upholstered for most of his career, like a bolster wearing a guru shirt. Rajendra Kumar … well, what can you say? And yet, these men were serious stars … Why does Indian cinema, deal in beautiful women and ugly men? … Indian cinema favours good-looking women and bad-looking men because its audiences consist of good-looking women and bad-looking men … Think about it: what choice do they have? In nearly every arranged marriage in North India you will hear an older woman say reassuringly: "*Ladkon ki seerat dekhi jaati hai, soorat nahin*", which, roughly translated, reads: you look at a boy's qualities, not his looks.' (2008: 16–17).

54. Sen, Ronojoy, 2015: 217.

55. See also excellent biography by Rajiv Vijayakar (2018) of the actor Dharmendra.

56. Tulsi Badrinath, *Madras, Chennai and the Self: Conversations with the City*, New Delhi: Pan Macmillan, 02–15: 156.

57. This is a common misconception, India is not, of course, a largely vegetarian country. See, for instance: https://thewire.in/food/india-food-eating-vegetarianism (visited 5-3-2020).

58. While the idea of a 'new India' is ubiquitously present in popular media and academic research, there are a few books which have specifically informed my analysis here: Jyotsna Kapur's (2013) *The Politics of Time and Youth in Brand India: Bargaining with Capital* (Delhi: Anthem Press); Anthony P. D'Costa's (2010) *A New India?: Critical Reflections in the Long Twentieth Century* (New York and London: Anthem Press); Sirpa Tenhunen and Minna Säävälä (2012) *An Introduction to*

*Changing India: Culture, Politics and Development* (London: Anthem Press); Adam Roberts, (2017) *Superfast Primetime Ultimate Nation: The Relentless Invention of Modern India* (London: Profile Books).

59. See Baas, 2009. 'The IT Caste. Of Love and Marriage in the IT Industry of Bangalore'. *South Asia: Journal of South Asian Studies,* 32: 2, 285-307.

60. This in itself is a matter of discussion of course. For those living on one to two dollars a day, upper-middle-class lives of the South Delhi or Bandra West variety can seem very elite.

61. One lakh is a hundred thousand.

62. See also *Metabolic Living* by Harris Solomon (2016).

63. 'Goonda' means hired thug.

64. There's a difference in opinion what exactly 'morya' means here. Some suggest that it references the saint Morya Gosavi, who was a well-known fourteenth-century devotee of the Lord. Pleased with his worship, as the story goes, he was granted the boon (or wish) that his name should always be associated with Ganesha. Others suggest that 'morya' is actually a splitting of the words 'mhora ya', which means 'come ahead' or 'be in front'. In my experience, devotees mainly interpreted the sentence in terms of it being an honorific way of welcoming their God and not necessarily something that was concretely translatable into English. Besides, although Mumbai is the capital of Maharashtra and the state's official language is Marathi, it is not a language shared by all in the city. Kishore, for instance, speaks Odia at home, while Vijay is more likely to converse in English and Hindi.

65. Dasgupta, 2014: 16, italics in the original.

66. Shaadi means wedding.

67. See the example described in the first chapter for starters.

68. Unlike Hollywood, Bollywood actors are usually referred to by their first name. It hints at a particular intimacy 'fans' feel for

their heroes and heroines that is much less pronounced in the West.

69. Bhakti poetry celebrates love for and devotion to specific Hindu gods. It originally emerged in the seventh century, and is considered a reformist trend in Hinduism, offering a more individual-focused notion of devotion and spirituality.

70. I discuss caste-relations in particular with reference to Jat and Gujjar men in much greater detail in chapter 5.

71. *Hindustan Times*, 12 October 2013.

72. An akhara is a traditional place of wrestling that often also comes with facilities for boarding, lodging and training.

73. Informants usually called me 'Michael' rather than 'Michiel'.

74. Director Sanjay Leela Bhansali also went on record to say that the reference to 'Rasleela' should not be interpreted as a reference to Lord Krishna.

75. Wacquant, 1995: 66.

76. Ibid.

77. MuscleMania promotes itself as one of the world's leading natural bodybuilding competitions. A relatively recent addition to the bodybuilding scene, it differentiates itself from more regular bodybuilding competitions in that it usually includes separate competitions for (actual) bodybuilding, sports modelling, swimwear, fitness, etc.

78. Crossley, 2006: 23.

79. Linder, 2007: 452.

80. Moore, 1997: 2.

81. Ibid.

82. See Besnier, 2012: 493 for a more detailed discussion.

83. Ibid: 449.

84. See also Baas, 2017 where I discuss this in greater detail.

85. Indian bodybuilders usually refer to the junior/aspiring bodybuilders they coach as their 'students'. These students frequently refer to their coaches as their teachers or gurus. It is

not uncommon for younger bodybuilders to honour their trainers by respectfully touching their feet.

86. NABBA stands for National Amateur Body-Builders' Association. Originally founded in the United Kingdom in 1950, it has since become a label that is often used to provide an official élan to competitions in India as well as elsewhere.

87. Bhattacharjee, 'Of Fake Mr Universe!', *The Shillong Times*, Letter to the Editor, 7 December 2017. http://theshillongtimes. com/2017/12/07/of-fake-mr-universe/ (visited 24-03-2020)

88. See here: http://theshillongtimes.com/2017/11/01/ meghalaya-cop-to-represent-india-in-world-body-building-meet/ (visited 17-02-2020).

89. I assume the author means 'champion' here.

90. Watt, 2016: 1927.

91. Ibid: 1921–22.

92. Simeon Panda has an Instagram following of six million plus and his page on Facebook boasts 5.8 million likes. Lazar Angelov counts nearly six million followers on Instagram and over fourteen million likes on Facebook (visited 23-04-2020).

93. Watt, 2016: 1.

94. Sandow's India trip is also discussed in David L. Chapman's (1994) book, *Sandow the Magnificent: Eugen Sandow and the Beginnings of Bodybuilding*. Chapter 7, 'Triumphs and Travels, 1901–7', 129–163.

95. Stokvis, 2006: 466.

96. Watt, 2016: 2.

97. Wedemeyer, 1994: 472.

98. See also Carden-Coyne, 1999.

99. Watt, 2016: 2.

100. Ibid: 3.

101. As discussed and quoted in Watt, 2016: 8, though plenty of texts on colonial India and (related) issues of masculinity have similarly touched upon Macaulay's words.

102. Budd, 1997: 81.

103. See also Osella and Osella, 2006: 5.

104. Alter, 2004: 509.

105. Ibid: 509–510.

106. See for instance Joseph Alter's work on Hindu militancy (1994); Thomas Blom Hansen's 1996 study 'Recuperating Masculinity: Hindu Nationalism, Violence and the Exorcising of the Muslim Other', *Critique of Anthropology*, Vol. 16, no. 2, 137–72. Or Anand Patwardhan's well-known documentary (1992) *Ram ke Naam* (In the Name of God).

107. See for instance https://www.indiatvnews.com/news/india/maratha-bodybuilder-flexes-his-muscles-before-bal-thackeray-5122.html (visited 22-05-2018).

108. No connection with the well-known gym chain 'Gold's Gym'.

109. Parshathy J. Nath, *The Hindu*, 'Palavakkam's love for body builders', 1 March 2017: http://www.thehindu.com/todays-paper/tp-features/tp-metroplus/palavakkams-love-for-body-builders/article17386018.ece (last visited 17-05-2018).

110. Oddly, this now stands for International Federation of Bodybuilding and Fitness.

111. ACE stands for American Council on Exercise.

112. See also their website: https://www.gcctraining.net/ (visited 19-02-2019).

113. Solomon, 2015: 177.

114. Ibid: 178.

115. IBEF does not provide source material information for the way they have calculated different growth scenarios of the Indian food market. Figures can be found here: http://www.ibef.org/industry/indian-food-industry.aspx (visited 06-12-2016).

116. Article can be found here: http://economictimes.indiatimes.com/industry/cons-products/food/organic-food-market-growing-at-25-30-awareness-still-low-government/articleshow/49379802.cms (visited 06-12-2016).

117. See here: http://www.euromonitor.com/sports-nutrition-in-india/report (visited 06-12-2016).
118. Kirana shops are small neighbourhood retail stores selling mainly everyday items. Although supermarkets are on the rise, the bulk of Indian groceries continue to be purchased at such shops.
119. CrossFit refers to a functional training routine which takes place in a 'box', as its members will put it. Such a box is usually a rather spartanly equipped workout space that is low on equipment, instead focusing on exercises that mimic how the body is used in day-to-day life.
120. This 'true middle India' seems to be conceptualised as consisting of 60 per cent of households by income, or 164 million households. See Jayaraman, 2017: 8–9.
121. Jayaraman, 2017: 8–9.
122. Ibid: 10.
123. Kapur, 2012: 50.
124. Ibid: 51–52.
125. Ibid: 253.
126. Ibid: 254; as we find out later on in the book, Hari does manage to pay off his debts and now lives a more stable and disciplined life.
127. de Souza, Kumar and Shastri, 2009: ix.
128. See for the full case study de Souza, Kumar and Shastri, 2009: 38–39.
129. Titus, 2015: 122.
130. Ibid: 124.
131. Ibid: 124–6
132. Ibid: 133.
133. *The Indian Express*, 'From road rage to sports rage and more—masculinities in modern India', 29 June 2017.
134. See Gill, Henwood and Mclean, 2005: 39.
135. Turner, 2000: 42; as also discussed in Gill, Henwood and Mclean, 2005: 39.

136. Gill, Henwood and Mclean, 2005: 40; see for further discussion Simon Winlow, *Badfellas: Crime, Tradition and New Masculinities*. Oxford: Berg Publishers, 2001, 98–9.

137. Gill, Henwood and Mclean, 2005: 40.

138. See for its initial conceptualisation R.W. Connell's influential study *Masculinities* (1995).

139. Lohan, 2010: 14.

140. See Monaghan, 2002b: 334–5

141. According to Butler, gendered behaviour is performative because of the desire of the subject in question to be taken to belong to a particular gender category (e.g. male or female). The connection between anatomical sex and gendered behaviour is, in a sense, not important in this.

142. See Beynon, 2002.

143. As discussed in David Buchbinder, *Men and Masculinities*. London: Routledge, 2013, 2010: 35.

144. Ibid.

145. Chopra, 2004: 37.

146. de Neve, 2004: 62.

147. Ibid: 65.

148. Monaghan, 2002a: 409.

149. Winlow, 2001: 103, see also Monaghan, 2002a: 409.

150. Monaghan draws on Maurice Merleau-Ponty's (1962) phenomenology of embodiment here.

151. Melnik et al, 2007; Voelcker et al, 2010.

152. See for a more extensive discussion of India's middle class, patterns of consumption and the impact on urban space Brosius, 2010 and Fernandes, 2006.

153. See for a more detailed study of exercise dependence Banberry, Groves and Biscomb, 2011: 1–18.

154. See Hatoum and Belle, 2004, with specific reference to the role the media plays; Drummond, 2010, for the increase in food related disorders among men in a western context; Marzano-Parisoli,

2012, who discusses this with specific reference to bodybuilding; Williams and Ricciardelli 2014 for the influence of social media.

155. See Olivardia, 2001; Harvey and Robinson, 2003; Brown and Graham, 2008; Fardouly and Vartanian, 2016.

156. Mumford and Choudry, 2000; Sarah Grogan, 2008.

157. Monaghan, 1999, 2001, 2002; Lenehan, 2003; Probert et al, 2007; Petrocelli et al, 2008.

158. Gerritsen, 2019.

159. Pope, Olivardia, Gruber and Borowiekcki, 1999: 65–72.

160. This poem appeared in *The Times of India* on 2 September 2018, as part of Akhil Katyal's column 'Poetic Licence'. It is also available here: https://blogs.timesofindia.indiatimes.com/voices/poetic-licence/ (visited 01-09-2018).

161. Competitions in the Delhi/NCR-region would often refer to bodybuilders in the singular as 'bodybuilder'.

162. For a short but insightful portrait of the city see Malvika Singh, 2013.

163. Gurgaon was officially renamed Gurugram in 2016, but the competition took place before that. The reason I continue to use Gurgaon elsewhere is to avoid confusion.

164. 'NCR' is increasingly employed as a 'colloquial' shorthand for Delhi and its various surrounding areas which are spread over three adjoining states: Haryana (Faridabad and Gurgaon), Rajasthan (Bharatpur) and Uttar Pradesh (Ghaziabad, Meerut and Noida).

165. See for a detailed exploration Brosius's (2010) seminal work. Dupont's (2011) article on Delhi's dream of becoming a global city is also relevant here. Seth Schindler (2014) discusses such ambitions by focusing on the (changing) relations between street hawkers and the new middle class.

166. Bhan, 2016: 47.

167. Ibid: 150.

168. I use caste and community rather interchangeably in this chapter,

as is also common practice in Indian media. While membership to communities such as the Gujjars and Jats is caste-based, not everything these communities do or stand for is always directly related to specific caste-related issues (e.g. arranged marriages, dietary restrictions or temple practices).

169. Occasionally such stories also make it into newspapers, such as in *The Times of India* on 28 March, 2018: 'Old wrestlers "fight" to keep legacy alive.' With a focus on Madurai, it says: 'Unlike earlier days, youngsters today join the school [akhara] for bodybuilding purposes. With only a few opting for wrestling, the sport at the school is limited to elderly wrestlers... Keeping in mind the waning demand for wrestling, the school's trust upgraded it into a gymnasium in 1990.' Available online: https://timesofindia.indiatimes.com/city/madurai/old-wrestlers-fight-to-keep-legacy-alive/articleshow/63495099.cms (visited 11-09-2018).

170. Officially known as the Dronacharya Award for Outstanding Coaches in Sports and Games, this is a sports coaching honour that is named after Drona, often referred to as Dronacharya or Guru Drona, a character from the Mahabharata. It is awarded annually by the Ministry of Youth Affairs and Sports.

171. See also Govinda, 2013.

172. Roy, 2011: 223–238.

173. Chatterji, 2015: viii.

174. Acharya et al, 2017: 3.

175. See for a critical take on Delhi's Master Plan, Sharan, Awadhendra. *In the City, Out of Place: Nuisance, Pollution, and Dwelling in Delhi, c. 1850–2000.* New Delhi: Oxford University Press, 2014.

176. Govinda, 2013.

177. Chatterji, 2015: 75.

178. Narain, 2017: 146

179. Ibid.

180. See for background Chatterji (2013), with its focus on the 'micro politics' of urban transformation within a context of globalisation, specifically focusing on the case of Gurgaon. The way such developments have impacted the local Yadav community is also discussed by Cowan, 2018a as well as Dubey 2018 (with reference to Ghaziabad and Noida). Furthermore, Narain (2009) discusses land acquisition-related issues with reference to farmland (formerly) owned by the Jat community.

181. See for the Jat community: Jeffrey, 2010: 910. In contrast, it is interesting to note Fernandes and Heller's (2006) three-tiered classification of the Indian middle classes here. According to them, first come the senior professionals and higher bureaucrats; second, rich farmers and the urban petite bourgeoisie; and third, poorly paid members of the salariat, such as nurses, clerks and teachers. Although they do not provide further detail on what constitutes rich farmers, one may assume what is meant here are the upper-caste land owners, such as the Thakurs, though it wouldn't be much of a stretch to include certain Jat farmers here as well. See: Fernandes, L. & Heller, P. 2006. 'Hegemonic aspirations: new middle-class politics and India's democracy in comparative perspective', *Critical Asian Studies* 38(4), 495–522.

182. Singh, 2011: 20.

183. 'The unrest in Delhi shows that caste issues still blight India.' *The Guardian*, by Priya Virmani, 24 February 16.

184. It led one of India's leading magazines *Open* to dedicate an article to the community's demands and aspirations titled 'The Unreasonable Jats' (1003–2017). Others who have taken a critical eye to 'Jat demands' and the background of their various struggles include Radhika Bhatia's analysis in the *Economic and Political Weekly* titled 'Jats and Reservations in Haryana' 16 April 2016; and Ashwini Deshpande and Rajesh Ramachandran's (2017) 'Dominant or Backward?: Political Economy of Demand for Quotas by Jats, Patels and Marathas.' *Economic and Political Weekly*, 13 May 2017.

185. 'Big, fat Gujjar weddings: Easy come, easy go.' *The Times of India*, 13 March 2011. Available online: https://timesofindia. indiatimes.com/home/sunday-times/deep-focus/Big-fat-Gujjar-weddings-Easy-come-easy-go/articleshow/7689163.cms (visited 4-09-2018).

186. 'The Gujars Of Delhi.' *Outlook*, 18 July 2007. Available online: https://www.outlookindia.com/website/story/the-gujars-of-delhi/235119 (visited 04-08-2018) See also: Aakash Joshi, 'Gujjar Reservation: What They Want, and Why.' *The Quint*, 28 May 2015.

187. Singh, 2011: 21.

188. Satendra Kumar, 'Ethnography of Youth Politics: Leaders, Brokers and Morality in a Provincial University in Western Uttar Pradesh'. *History and Sociology of South Asia* 6(1), 2011: 41–70.

189. Govinda, 2013.

190. Ibid: 4.

191. Ajoy Ashirwad Mahaprashasta, 'Land and caste'. *Frontline*, 19 May–1 June 2012. Available online: https://www.frontline. in/static/html/fl2910/stories/20120601291010500.htm (visited 04-09-2018).

192. See: *The Indian Express* (30 April 2014), 'Noida village simmers after Gujjars and Dalits clash.' https://indianexpress.com/article/cities/delhi/noida-village-simmers-after-Gujjars-and-dalits-clash/ (visited 04-09-2018). And *The Pioneer*, 'Youth Dies as Gujjars, Jatavs Fire 150 rounds.' 29 April 2014. https://www.dailypioneer.com/todays-newspaper/youth-dies-as-Gujjars-jatavs-fire-150-rounds.html (visited 04-09-2018).

193. There's a law that requires 25 per cent of a plot of land to have been built on so as to guarantee continued ownership. A common practice in the Greater Noida region is to build some basic structure of bricks to meet this requirement and prevent the government seizing the land as unused.

194. See for further details: Pankaj Bhatia, 'On Delhi's outskirts,

violence over real estate, not caste.' *Governance Now*, 26 May 2015. Available here: https://www.governancenow.com/news/regular-story/delhis-outskirts-violence-over-real-estate-not-caste (05-10-2018).

195. 'Sh.' stands for Shri, or honourable.

196. See here: https://www.youtube.com/watch?v=WfWg2dfA7gQ (visited 20-02-2019).

197. Chiku, chikoo or sapodilla is known as an energy-boosting food because it is loaded with fructose and sucrose. It is believed to have various other health benefits, rooted in ayurvedic thinking.

198. Sengupta, 2016: 16.

199. A fragment from the original poem titled 'I Sing the Body Electric' (1855), which first appeared without this title in Whitman's *Leaves of Grass*. The book's 1867 edition mentions the title for the first time. The full text can also be found here: https://www.poetryfoundation.org/poems/45472/i-sing-the-body-electric (accessed 22-04-2020).

200. Please note that I have referred to this informant as Kishore in another publication (Baas, 2017). In order to prevent confusion with the Kishore who featured in chapter one and six, I will refer to him as Girish here. Kishore as well as Girish are pseudonyms, of course.

201. Please note that the quotes that I am using here are those from the English-language subtitles (the actors speak primarily in Hindi).

202. Shefalee Vasudev, 'The New Second Sex. Exploited, Underpaid, Underemployed, and Still Dreaming, the Agony of the Indian Male Model', *Open*, 4 December 2017: 20–29.

203. Ibid: 23.

204. Ibid: 24.

205. Ibid: 26.

206. Ibid: 24.

207. Ibid: 27.

208. Rohit K. Dasgupta analyses this in 'The Queer Rhetoric of Bollywood: A Case of Mistaken Identity', http://interalia.org.pl/ index_pdf.php?lang=en&klucz=&produkt=1353788763-695 (visited 17-04-2019).

209. See here: https://www.firstpost.com/entertainment/ gunday-review-its-all-about-ranveer-singh-and-arjun-kapoors-bromance-1390339.html (visited 17-04-2019).

210. See here: https://www.firstpost.com/entertainment/ padmaavat-amid-rajput-romance-and-valour-bhansali-gives-us-a-most-queer-love-story-4333679.html (visited 17-04-2019).

211. In a 2009 article in *The Guardian*, we read the following: '*Men's Health* does not take kindly to having its sexuality questioned; as an ex-staffer told me: "There's total bewilderment over there the gay thing. And yet look at it! It's high camp, isn't it?" The *Men's Health* men do indeed respond with bewilderment and a degree of crossness to the gay question: "There are lots of great gay titles out there," says Mike Shallcross firmly; "*Men's Health* is *not* one of them." ("I just don't get the gay thing," adds Toby Wiseman. "I mean, what's gay about *those* bodies? Skinny androgynous boys in fashion shoots in other magazines—surely *that's* much more gay?")' https://www.theguardian.com/ lifeandstyle/2009/sep/27/magazines (visited 17-04-2019).

212. Chapman, 2013: 193.

213. Ibid: 9–10.

214. Alvarez, 2008: 48–49.

215. Ibid: 50.

216. See also Ibid: 57.

217. Boyle, 2010: 156, drawing on Pronger, 1990.

218. Alter, 2005: 47.

219. Ibid: 48. The discussion of the term is long and varied. It can mean excellent of any kind, but has also been held to refer to moral virtue. It sometimes points at an understanding of virtue as (human) knowledge, the highest human potential, etc.

220. E.g. Whitehead, 2002; Hearn, 2004; Lohan, 2010. I am obviously making significant shortcuts here, but the gist of the argument does follow this type of reasoning. I am not necessarily critical of the studies that genuinely sought to argue for such a crisis but argue that it's not an easy argument to transplant to the Indian case, even if it may seem that India with its patriarchal gender relations and violence against women makes for a 'perfect' case here.

221. Richardson, 2004: 50

222. Sengupta, 2016: 141.

223. An important exercise to build strength for wrestlers, involving jori or clubs of various sizes which are swung in a variety of ways over and around the body.

224. Alter, 2005: 47–60.

225. Richardson, 2004: 53.

226. Ibid.

227. Baas, 2017: 10–11.

# BIBLIOGRAPHY

## BOOKS

Acharya, Sanghmitra S., Sucharita Sen, Milap Punia and Sunita Reddy. 'Land, Livelihoods and Health: Marginalization in Globalizing Delhi'. In *Marginalization in Globalizing Delhi: Issues of Land, Livelihoods and Health*, edited by Sanghmitra S. Acharya, Sucharita Sen, Milap Punia and Sunita Reddy, 1-18. India: Springer, 2017.

Alexander, Susan M. 'Stylish Hard Bodies: Branded Masculinity in "Men's Health" Magazine'. *Sociological Perspectives*, 46, no. 4 (2003): 535–54.

Alter, Joseph S. *The Wrestler's Body*. Berkeley, Los Angeles, Oxford: University of California Press, 1992.

Alvarez, Erick. *Muscle Boys: Gay Gym Culture*. New York and London: Routledge, 2008.

Anand, Dibyesh. 'The Violence of Security: Hindu Nationalism and the Politics of Representing "the Muslim" as a Danger'. *The Round Table*, 94, no. 379 (2005): 203–15.

Anand, Dibyesh. 'Anxious Sexualities: Masculinity, Nationalism and Violence'. *BJPIR*, 9, no. 2 (2007): 257–69.

Andreasson, Jesper. '"Shut Up and Squat!" Learning Body Knowledge within the Gym'. *Ethnography and Education*, 9, no. 1 (2014): 1–15.

Anshuman, Kumar. 'The Unreasonable Jats.' *Open*, 10 March 2017. http://www.openthemagazine.com/article/politics/the-unreasonable-jats.

Atkinson, Michael. 'Playing with Fire: Masculinity, Health, and Sports Supplements.' *Sociology of Sport Journal*, 24 (2007): 165–86.

Atkinson, Michael. 'Masks of Masculinity: (Sur)passing Narratives and Cosmetic Surgery.' In *Body/Embodiment: Symbolic Interaction and the Sociology of the Body*, edited by Dennis Waskul and Phillip Vannini, 247–61. England: Ashgate, 2006.

Attwood, Fiona. ''Tits and Ass and Porn and Fighting': Male Heterosexuality in Magazines for Men.' *International Journal of Cultural Studies*, 8 (2005): 83–100.

Azzarito, Laura. 'The Rise of the Corporate Curriculum: Fatness, Fitness, and Whiteness.' In *Biopolitics and the 'Obesity Epidemic': Governing Bodies*, edited by Jan Wright and Valerie Harwood, 183–96. New York & London: Routledge, 2009.

Banbery, Stuart, Mark Groves, and Kay Biscomb. 'The Relationship between Exercise Dependence and Identity Reinforcement: A Sociological Examination of a Gym-based Environment in the United Kingdom.' *Sport in Society*, 15, no. 9 (2012): 1242–59.

Banerjee, Sikata. 'Introduction: Constructs of Nation and Gender.' In *Make Me a Man!: Masculinity, Hinduism, and Nationalism in India*, edited by Harold Coward, 1–19. Albany: State University of New York, 2005.

Badrinath, Tulsi. *Madras, Chennai and the Self: Conversations with the City*. New Delhi: Pan Macmillan, 2015.

Banke, Ingo J., Peter M. Prodinger, Simone Waldt, Gregor Weirich, Boris M. Holzapfel, Reiner Gradinger, and Hans Rechl. 'Irreversible Muscle Damage in Bodybuilding due to Long-Term Intramuscular Oil Injection.' *International Journal of Sports Medicine*, 33, no. 10 (2012): 829–34.

Beegom, Raheena, Razia Beegom, Mohammad a. Niaz, and Ram B. Singh. 'Diet, Central Obesity and Prevalence of Hypertension in the Urban Population of South India.' *International Journal of Cardiology*, 51, no. 2 (1995): 183–91.

Belliappa, Jyothsna Latha. 'Setting Out to Study Class and Gender in Contemporary India.' In *Gender, Class and Reflexive Modernity in India*, pp. 1–21. England: Palgrave Macmillan, 2013.

Belliappa, Jyothsna Latha. 'Conclusion: The Collective Project of Self.' In *Gender, Class and Reflexive Modernity in India*, 160–6. England: Palgrave Macmillan, 2013.

Besnier, Niko. 'The Athelete's Body and the Global Condition: Tongan Rugby Players in Japan.' *American Ethnologist*, 39, no. 3 (2012): 491–510.

Besnier, Niko and Susan Brownell. 'Sport, Modernity, and the Body.' *Annual Review of Anthropology*, 41 (2012): 443–59.

Bhan, Gautam. *In the Public's Interest. Evictions, Citizenship and Inequality in Contemporary Delhi*. Hyderabad: Orient BlackSwan, 2016.

Bhatt, Amy, Madhavi Murty and Priti Ramamurthy. 'Hegemonic Developments: The New Indian Middle Class, Gendered Subalterns, and Diasporic Returnees in the Event of Neoliberalism.' *Signs*, 36, no. 1 (2010): 127–52.

Bhattacharjee. 'Of Fake Mr Universe!' *The Shillong Times*, Letter to the Editor, 7 December 2017.

Bourdieu, Pierre (trans. Nice, R.). *Distinction: A Social Critique of the Judgement of Taste*. Cambridge: Harvard University Press, 1984.

Bourdieu, Pierre (trans. Nice, R.). *Outline of a Theory of Practice*. Cambridge: Cambridge University Press, 1978.

Boyle, Ellexis. 'Marketing muscular masculinity in Arnold: The Education of a Bodybuilder.' *Journal of Gender Studies*, 19, no. 2 (2010): 153–66.

Brod, Harry and Kaufman, Michael (eds.). *Masculinity as Homophobia: Fear, Shame and Silence in the Construction of Gender Identity*. Newbury Park: Sage Publications, 1994.

Brown, Jac and Doug Graham. 'Body Satisfaction in Gym-active

Males: An Exploration of Sexuality, Gender, and Narcissm.' *Sex Roles*, 59 (2008): 94–106.

Brosius, Christiane. *India's Middle Class: New Forms of Urban Leisure, Prosperity and Consumption*. New Delhi: Routledge, 2010.

Bruckert, Michaël. 'Changing Food Habits in Contemporary India: Discourses and Practices from the Middle Classes in Chennai (Tamil Nadu).' In *Routledge Handbook of Contemporary India*, edited by Knut A. Jacobsen, 457–73. New York: Routledge, 2015.

Budd, Michael Anton. 'Imperial Mirrors.' In *The Sculpture Machine: Physical Culture and Body Politics in the Age of Empire*, pp. 81–100. Hampshire & London: Macmillan Press Ltd, 1997.

Butler, Judith. *Gender Trouble: Feminism and the Subversion of Identity*. 2nd ed. London and New York: Routledge, 1999.

Caplan, Pat. 'Crossing the Veg/Non-Veg Divide: Commensality and Sociality among the Middle Classes in Madras/Chennai.' *South Asia: Journal of South Asian Studies*, 31, no. 1 (2008): 118–42.

Carden-Coyne, Anna Alexandra. 'Classical Heroism and Modern Life: Bodybuilding and Masculinity in the Early Twentieth Century.' *Journal of Australian Studies*, 23, no. 63 (1999): 138–49.

Chakraborty, Chandrima. *Masculinity, Asceticism, Hinduism: Past and Present Imaginings of India*. Ranikhet (India): Permanent Black, 2011.

Chapman, David L. 'Triumphs and Travels 1901–7.' In *Sandow the Magnificent: Eugen Sandow and the Beginnings of Bodybuilding*, pp. 129–163. Urbana & Chicago: University of Illinois Press, 1994.

Chapman, David L. *Universal Hunks. A Pictorial History of Muscular Men Around the World*, 1895–1975. Vancouver: Asenal Pulp Press, 2013.

Chatterji, Tathagata. *Citadels of Glass. The Story of India's New Suburban Landscape*. Chennai: westland ltd., 2015.

Chatterji, Tathagata. 'The Micro-Politics of Urban Transformation in the Context of Globalisation: A Case Study of Gurgaon, India.' *South Asia: Journal of South Asian Studies*, 36, no. 2 (2013): 273–87.

Correspondent, 'Body Building: Jagtar Adjudged Mr Libra 2017.' *The Tribune*, 31 December 2017.

Correspondent, 'Hoshairpur's Bunty Adjudged Mr North India.' *The Tribune*, 30 October 2017.

Cowan, Thomas. 'The Urban Village, Agrarian Transformation, and Rentier Capitalism in Gurgaon, India.' *Antipode*, 50, no. 5 (2018): 1244–66.

Cowan, Thomas. 'Subaltern Counter-urbanism: Work, Dispossession and Emplacement in Gurgaon, India.' *Geoforum*, 92 (2018): 152–60.

Crossley, Nick. 'In the Gym: Motives, Meaning and Moral Careers.' *Body & Society*, 12, no. 3 (2006): 23–50.

Crossley, Nick. 'The Networked Body and the Question of Reflexivity.' In *Body/Embodiment: Symbolic Interaction and the Sociology of the Body*, edited by Dennis Waskul and Phillip Vannini, 21–33. England: Ashgate, 2006.

Culbertson, Philip. 'Designing Men: Reading the Male Body as Text.' *The Journal of Textual Reasoning*, 7, no. 1 (1998), online only (no page numbers): http://jtr.shanti.virginia.edu/designing-men-reading-the-male-body-as-text/.

Dabral, Shweta and S.L. Malik. 'Demographic Study of Gujjars of Delhi: I. Population Structure and Socio-cultural Profile.' *Journal of Human Ecology*, 16, no. 1 (2004): 17–24.

Dasgupta, Parasmani, Rana Saha, and Maarten Nubé. 'Changes in Body Size, Shape and Nutritional Status of Middle-Class Bengali Boys of Kolkata, India, 1982-2002.' *Economics and Human Biology*, 6, no. 1 (2008): 75–94.

Dasgupta, Rana. *Capital. A Portrait of Twenty-First Century Delhi*. New Delhi: Fourth Estate, 2014.

Datta, Damayanti. 'The Booby Trap.' *India Today*, 30 April 2012.

Deepa, M., S. Farooq, R. Deepa, D. Manjula, and V. Mohan. 'Prevalence and Significance of Generalized and Central Body Obesity in an Urban Asian Indian Population in Chennai, India (CURES:

47).' *European Journal of Clinical Nutrition*, 63, no. 2 (2009): 259–67.

Demerath III, N.J., Surinder S. Jodhka, and Loren R. Demerath. 'Interrogating Caste and Religion in India's Emerging Middle Class.' *Economic & Political Weekly*, 41, no. 35 (2006): 3813–8.

Deshpande, Ashwini and Rajesh Ramachandran. 'Dominant or Backward?: Political Economy of Demad for Quotas by Jats, Patels, and Marathas.' *Economic & Political Weekly*, 52, no. 19 (2016): 8–90.

Dickey, Sara. 'The Pleasures and Anxieties of Being in the Middle: Emerging Middle-Class Identities in Urban South India.' *Modern Asian Studies*, 46, no. 3 (2012): 559–99.

Dittrich, Christoph. 'The Changing Food Scenario and the Middle Classes in the Emerging Megacity of Hyderabad, India.' In *The New Middle Classes: Globalizing Lifestyles, Consumerism and Environmental Concern*, edited by Hellmuth Lange and Lars Meier, 269–80. Dordrecht & New York: Springer, 2009.

Diwekar, Rujuta. *Don't Lose Your Mind, Lose Your Weight*. New Delhi: Random House India, 2009.

Donner, Henrike and Geert De Neve. 'Introduction.' In *Being Middle-class in India: A Way of Life*, edited by Henrike Donner, 1–22. New York: Routledge, 2011.

Dua, Rachit. 'Amidst Recurring Financial Troubles, Junaid Kaliwala Created History in Bodybuilding.' *The Logical Indian*, 1 November 2017.

Dubey, Shruti. 'Urban Transformations in Khora Village, NCR: A View from the "Periphery".' *Economic & Political Weekly*, 53, no. 12 (2018): 76–84.

Dupont, Véronique D.N. 'The Dream of Delhi as a Global City.' *International Journal of Urban and Regional Research*, 35, no. 3 (2011): 533–54.

Edgley, Charles. 'The Fit and Healthy Body: Consumer Narratives and the Management of Postmodern Corporeity.' In *Body/Embodiment:*

*Symbolic Interaction and the Sociology of the Body,* edited by Dennis Waskul and Phillip Vannini, 231–45. England: Ashgate, 2006.

Fardouly, Jasmine and Lenny R. Vartanian. 'Social Media and the Body Image Concerns: Current Research and Future Directions.' *Current Opinion in Psychology,* 9 (2016): 1–5.

FPJ News Service. 'Ujjain: City Youths Win Prizes in Divisional Body Building Championship.' *The Free Press Journal,* 30 December 2017.

Friedman, Sam. 'The Price of the Ticket: Rethinking the Experience of Social Mobility.' *Sociology,* 48, no. 2 (2014): 352–68.

Fuller, C.J., and Haripriya Narasimhan. 'Information Technology Professionals and the New-rich Middles Class in Chennai.' *Modern Asian Studies,* 41, no. 1 (2007): 121–50.

Garber, M. 'Fetish Envy.' *October,* 54 (1990): 45–55.

Giardino, Joseph C. and Mary E. Procidano. 'Muscle Dysmorphia Symptomatology: A Cross-Cultural Study in Mexico and the United States.' *International Journal of Men's Health,* 11, no. 1 (2012): 83–103.

Giazitzoglu, Andreas. 'Qualitative Upward Mobility, the Mass-Media and "Posh" Masculinity in Contemporary North-East Britain: A Micro Sociological Case-Study.' *Sociological Research Online,* 19, no. 2 (2014). https://journals.sagepub.com/doi/full/10.5153/sro.3273.

Gill, Rosalind, Karen Henwood, and Car; McLean. 'Body Projects and the Regulation of Normative Masculinity.' *Body & Society,* 11, no. 1 (2005): 37–62.

Gooptu, Nandini. 'Neoliberal Subjectivity, Enterprise Culture and New Workplaces: Organised Retail and Shopping Malls in India.' *Economic & Political Weekly,* 44, no. 22 (2009): 45–54.

Govinda, Radhika. 'First Our Fields, Now our Women': Gender Politics in Delhi's Urban Villages in Transition.' *South Asia Multidisciplinary Academic Journal,* 8 (2013): 1–15. https://journals.openedition.org/samaj/3648.

Greenhalgh, Susan. 'Weighty Subjects: The Biopolitics of the U.S. War on Fat.' *American Ethnologist*, 39, no. 3 (2012): 471–87.

Grogan, Sarah. 2008. *Body Image: Understanding Body Dissatisfaction in Men, Women and Children*, London & New York: Routledge.

Gupta, Dipankar. *Interrogating Caste. Understanding Hierarchy & Difference in Indian Society*. New Delhi: Penguin, 2000.

Halse, Christine. 'Bio-Citizenship: Virtue Discourses and the Birth of the Bio-Citizen.' In *Biopolitics and the 'Obesity Epidemic': Governing Bodies*, edited by Jan Wright and Valerie Harwood, 45–59. New York & London: Routledge, 2009.

Hansen, Thomas Blom. 'Recuperating Maculinity: Hindu Nationalism, Violence and the Exorcism of the Muslim "Other".' *Critique of Anthropology*, 16, no. 2 (1996): 137–72.

Harriss, John. 'Middle-Class Activism and the Politics of the Informal Working Class.' *Critical Asian Studies*, 38, no. 4 (2006): 445–65.

Harvey, Jeffery A. and John D. Robinson. 'Eating Disorders in Men: Current Considerations.' *Journal of Clinical Psychology in Medical Settings*, 10, no. 4 (2003): 297–306.

Harwood, Valerie. 'Theorizing Biopedagogies.' In *Biopolitics and the 'Obesity Epidemic': Governing Bodies*, edited by Jan Wright and Valerie Harwood, 15–30. New York & London: Routledge, 2009.

Jeffrey, Craig. 'Great Expectations. Youth in Contemporary India.' In *A Companion to the Anthropology of India*, edited by Isabelle Clark- Decès, 62–79. Malden, MA: Wiley-Blackwell, 2011.

Hatoum, Ida Jodette and Deborah Belle. 'Mags and Abs: Media Consumption and Bodily concerns in Men.' *Sex Roles*, 51, no. 7/8 (2004): 397–407.

Hess, Alex. 'Brawn Again: Why Hollywood's Muscle Heroes are Bigger than Ever.' *The Guardian*, 18 September 2018.

Indian Body Builders Federation. '10 Mr. India 2017: National Bodybuilding & Physique Sports Championship.' *Flyer*, 2–4 March 2017.

Jain, Kajri. 'Muscularity and its Ramifications: Mimetic Male Bodies in Indian Mass Culture.' *South Asia: Journal of South Asian Studies,* 24 (2001): 198–224.

Jain, Rimjhim. 'From Road Rage to Sports Rage and More—Masculinities in Modern India.' *The Indian Express,* 29 June 2017.

Jayadeva, Sazana. 'Below English Line': An Ethnographic Exploration of Class and the English Language in Post-liberalization India.' *Modern Asian Studies,* 52, no. 2 (2018): 576–608.

Jeffrey, Craig. 'Kicking Away the Ladder: Student Politics and the Making of an Indian Middle Class.' *Environment and Planning D: Society and Space,* 26 (2008): 517–36.

Jeffrey, Craig. ''Generation Nowhere': Rethinking Youth through the Lens of Unemployed Young Men.' *Progress in Human Geography,* 32, no. 6 (2008): 739–58.

Jeffrey, Craig. 'Kicking Away the Ladder: Student Politics and the Making of an Indian Middle Class.' *Internationales Asienforum,* 41, no. 1–2 (2010): 5–31.

Jeffrey, Craig. 'Timepass: Youth, Class, and Time among Unemployed Young Men in India.' *American Ethnologist,* 37, no. 3 (2010): 465–81.

Joshi, Sanjay. *Fractured Modernity: Making of a Middle Class in Colonial North India.* New Delhi: Oxford University Press, 2001.

Kapoor, Deepti. 'Driving in Greater Noida.' *Granta Magazine,* 23 February 2015.

Kelly, Tamara, Woo-ick Yang, C-S Chen, Kristen Reynolds, and Jiang He. 'Global Burden of Obesity in 2005 and Projections to 2030.' *International Journal of Obesity,* 32 (2008): 1431–7.

Kesavan, Mukul. *The Ugliness of the Indian Male and Other Propositions.* Ranikhet: Black Kite, 2008.

Kharas, Homi. 'The Emerging Middle Class in Developing Countries.' OECD Development Centre, Paris, *Working Paper No. 285,* January 2010.

Klein, Alan. M. *Little Big Men. Bodybuilding Subculture and Gender Construction.* Albany: State University of New York Press, 1993.

Kochhar, Rajesh. 'Denationalised Middle Class: Global Escape from Mandal.' *Economic & Political Weekly*, 39, no. 1 (2004): 20.

Krishnaswamy, Kamala, ed. *Obesity in the Urban Middle Class in Delhi.* Delhi: Nutrition Foundation of India, 1998.

Kulkarni, V.G. 'Marketing: The Middle-Class Bulge.' *Far Eastern Economic Review*, 156, no. 2 (1993): 44–6.

Kumar, Radhika. 'Stooping to Conquer: Jats and Reservations in Haryana.' *Economic & Political Weekly*, 51, no. 16 (2016): 15–18.

LaDousa, Chaise. *Hindi is Our Ground, English is Our Sky. Education, Language, and Social Class in Contemporary India.* New York: Berghahn Book, 2016.

Lakha, Salim. 'The State, Globalisation and Indian Middle-Class Identity.' In *Culture and Privilege in Capitalist Asia*, edited by Michael Pinches, 251–74. London: Routledge, 1999.

Lange, Hellmuth and Lars Meier. 'Who are the New Middle Classes and Why Are They Given So Much Public Attention.' In *The New Middle Classes: Globalizing Lifestyles, Consumerism and Environmental Concern*, edited by Hellmuth Lange and Lars Meier, 1–28. Dordrecht & New York: Springer, 2009.

Lange, Hellmuth, Lars Meier, and N.S. Anuradha. 'Highly Qualified Employees in Bangalore, India: Consumerist Predators?' In *The New Middle Classes: Globalizing Lifestyles, Consumerism and Environmental Concern*, edited by Hellmuth Lange and Lars Meier, 281–98. Dordrecht & New York: Springer, 2009.

Leahy, Deana. 'Disgusting Pedagogies.' In *Biopolitics and the 'Obesity Epidemic': Governing Bodies*, edited by Jan Wright and Valerie Harwood, 172–82. New York & London: Routledge, 2009.

Lenehan, Pat. *Anabolic Steroids and Other Performance-enhancing Drugs.* London & New York: Taylor & Francis, 2003.

Linder, Fletcher. 'Life as Art, and Seeing the Promise of Big Bodies.' *American Ethnologist*, 34, no. 3 (2007): 451–72.

Lokohare, Madhura. 'Iconographies of Urban Masculinity: Reading "Flex Boards" in an Indian City.' *Asia Pacific Perspectives*, 15, no. 1

(Fall 2017). https://www.usfca.edu/center-asia-pacific/perspectives/v15n1/lohokare.

Mahaprashasta, Ajoy Ashirwad. 'Land and Caste.' *Frontline*, 29, no. 10, 19 May–1 June 2012. https://frontline.thehindu.com/static/html/fl2910/stories/20120601291010500.htm.

Mainardi, Robert. *Strong Men: Vintage Photos of a Masculine Icon*. Chicago: Council Oak Books, 2001.

Marzano-Parisoli, Maria Michela. 'The Contemporary Construction of a Perfect Body Image: Bodybuilding, Exercise Addiction, and Eating Disorders. *Quest*, 52, no. 3 (2001): 216–30.

Mawdsley, Emma. 'India's Middles classes and the Environment.' *Development and Change*, 35, no. 1 (2004): 79–103.

Melnik, Bodo, Thomas Jansen, Stephan Grabbe. 'Abuse of Anabolic-androgenic Steroids and Bodybuilding Acne: An Underestimated Health Problem.' *Journal of the German Society of Dermatology*, 5, no. 2 (2007): 110–7.

Meyer, Christian and Nancy Birdsall. *New Estimates of India's Middle Class*. Technical Note. Washington, D.C.: Centre for Global Development, Peterson Institute for International Economics, November 2012.

Midha, Tanu, Bhola Nath, Ranjeeta Kumari, Yashwant Kumar Rao and Umeshwar Pandey. 'Childhood Obesity in India: A Meta-Analysis.' *The Indian Journal of Pediatrics*, 79, no. 7 (2012): 945–8.

Mokani, Paresh. 'Joel Gonsalves Sets the Tone.' *The Times of India*, 19 June 2017.

Monaghan, Lee. 'Challenging Medicine? Bodybuilding, Drugs and Risk.' *Sociology of Health & Illness*, 21, no. 6 (1999): 707–34.

Monaghan, Lee F. 'Vocabularies of Motive for Illicit Steroid Use among Bodybuilders.' *Social Science & Medicine*, 55 (2002): 695–708.

Monaghan, Lee F. 'Big Handsome Men, Bears and Others: Virtual Constructions of "Fat Male Embodiment".' *Body & Society*, 11, no. 2 (2005): 81–111.

Monaghan, Lee F. 'Body Mass Index, Masculinities and Moral Worth: Men's Critical Understandings of "Appropriate" Weight-for-height.' *Sociology of Health & Illness*, 29, no. 4 (2007): 584–609.

Monaghan, Lee F. *Bodybuilding, Drugs and Risk*. London & New York: Routledge, 2001.

Monaghan, Lee F. *Men and the War on Obesity: A Sociological Study*. London & New York: Routledge, 2008.

Monaghan, Lee F. 'McDonaldizing Men's Bodies? Slimming, Associated (Ir)Rationalities and Resistances.' *Body & Society*, 13, no. 2 (2007): 67–93.

Monaghan, Lee F. 'Men, Physical Activity, and the Obesity Discourse: Critical Understandings from a Qualitative Study.' *Sociology of Sport Journal*, 25 (2008): 97–129.

Mulvey, Christopher. 'Male Bodybuilding: Theorizing the Hyperbuilt Body.' Unpublished essay, winner of the Yale GALA Senior Essay Award, 2015.

Mumford, David Bardwell and Iffat Yaqub Choudry. 'Body Dissatisfaction and Eating Attitudes in Slimming and Fitness Gyms in London and Lahore: A Cross-Cultural Study.' *European Eating Disorders Review*, 8 (2000): 217–24.

Murphy, Jonathan. 'Indian Call Centre Workers: Vanguard of a Global Middle Class.' *Work, Employment & Society*, 25, no. 3 (2011): 417–33.

Murray, Samantha. 'Marked as "Pathological": "Fat" Bodies as Virtual Confessors.' In *Biopolitics and the 'Obesity Epidemic': Governing Bodies*, edited by Jan Wright and Valerie Harwood, 78–90. New York & London: Routledge, 2009.

Murray, Samantha. 'Pathologizing 'Fatness': Medical Authority and Popular Culture.' *Sociology of Sport Journal*, 25 (2008): 7–21.

Narain, Vishal. 'Growing City, Shrinking Hinterland: Land Acquisition, Transition, and Conflict in Peri-urban Gurgaon, India.' *Environment & Urbanization*, 21, no. 2 (2009): 501–12.

Narain, Vishal. 'Taken for a Ride? Mainstreaming Periurban Transport with Urban Expansion Policies.' *Land Use Policy*, 64 (2017): 145–52.

Nath, Parshathy J. 'Palavakkam's Love for Body Builders.' *The Hindu*, 1 March 2017.

Nijman, Jan. 'Mumbai's Mysterious Middle Class.' *International Journal of Urban and Regional Research*, 30. No. 4 (2006): 758–75.

Olivardia, Roberto. 'Mirror, Mirror on the Wall, Who's the Largest of Them All? The Features and Phenomenology of Muscle Dysmorphia.' *Harvard Review of Psychiatry*, 9, no. 5 (2001): 254–9.

Petrocelli, Matthew, Trish Oberweis, and Joseph Petrocelli. 'Getting Huge, Getting Ripped: A Qualitative Exploration of Recreational Steroid Use.' *Journal of Drug Issues*, 38, no. 4 (2008): 1187–205.

Pompper, Donnalyn. 'Masculinities, the Metrosexual, and Media Images: Across Dimensions of Age and Ethnicity.' *Sex Roles*, 63 (2010): 682–96.

Poonam, Snigdha. *Dreamers. How Young Indians Are Changing the World*. London: Hurst & Company, 2018.

Probert, Anne, Farah Palmer and Sarah Leberman. 'The Fine Line: An Insight into 'Risky' Practices of Male and Female Competitive Bodybuilders.' *Annals of Leisure Research*, 10, no. 3–4 (2007): 272–90.

Pronger, Brian. *The Arena of Masculinity: Sport, Homosexuality and the Meaning of Sex*. Toronto: University of Toronto Press, 1990.

Radhakrishnan, Smitha. 'Examining the 'Global' Indian Middle Class: Gender and Culture in the Silicon Valley/Bangalore Circuit.' *Journal of Intercultural Studies*, 29, no. 1 (2008): 7–20.

Ramachandran, A., C. Snehalatha, R. Vinitha, Megha Thayyil, C.K. Sathish Kumar, L. Sheeba, S. Joseph, and V. Vijay. 'Prevalence of Overweight in Urban Indian Adolescent School Children.' *Diabetes Research and Clinical Practice*, 57, no. 3 (2002): 185–90.

Ramesh, P.R. 'Out to Bait the Middle Class', *Open*, 3 February 2014.

Rawle, Tom. 'Welcome to the Small Village that is the Bodybuilding

Capital of the World.' *Daily Star*, video, 29 June 2014. https://www.dailystar.co.uk/diet-fitness/386364/Welcome-to-the-small-village-that-is-the-bodybuilding-capital-of-the-world.

Reporter. 'Vision of the Future: Sheru Aangrish.' *Fitness Guru*, 1, no. 3, October 2013.

Ricciardelli, Rosemary, Kimberley A. Clow, and Philip White. 'Investigating Hegemonic Masculinity: Portrayals of Masculinity in Men's Lifestyle Magazines.' *Sex Roles*, 63 (2010): 64–78.

Richardson, Niall. 'The Queer Activity of Extreme Male Bodybuilding: Gender Dissidence, Auto-eroticism and Hysteria.' *Social Semiotics*, 14, no. 1 (2004): 49–65.

Rogers, Martyn. 'Modernity, 'Authenticity', and Ambivalence: Subaltern Masculinities on a South Indian College Campus.' *Journal of the Royal Anthropological Institute*, 14, no. 1 (2008): 79–95.

Roy, Devapriya. *The Weight Loss Club. The Curious Experiments of Nancy Housing Cooperative*. New Delhi: Rupa Publications, 2013.

Roy, Parama. 'Meat-Eating, Masculinity, and renunciation in India: A Gandhian Grammar of Diet.' *Gender & History*, 14, no. 1 (2002): 62–91.

Rutten, Mario. 'Gujarat Earthquake in Wider Perspective. Involvement and Indifference.' *Economic & Political Weekly*, 36, no. 35 (2001): 3358–61.

Sanders, Clinton R. 'Viewing the Body: An Overview, Exploration and Extension.' In *Body/Embodiment: Symbolic Interaction and the Sociology of the Body*, edited by Dennis Waskul and Phillip Vannini, 279-94. England: Ashgate, 2006.

Säävälä, Minna. 'Entangled in the Imagination: New Middle-Class Apprehensions in an Indian Theme Park.' *Ethnos*, 71, no. 3 (2006): 390–414.

Schindler, Seth. 'The Making of "World-Class" Delhi: Relations between Street Hawkers and the New Middle Class.' *Antipode*, 46, no. 2 (2014): 557–73.

Sen, Ronojoy. *Nation at Play: A History of Sport in India*. New York: Columbia University Press. 2015, p. 217.

Sengupta, Rudraneil. *Enter the Dangal. Travels through India's Wrestling Landscape*. Noida: Harper Sport, 2016.

Sengupta, Somini. *The End of Karma. Hope and Fury among India's Youth*. New Delhi: HarperCollins, 2016.

Sharan, Awadhendra. *In the City, Out of Place. Nuisance, Pollution, and Dwelling in Delhi, c. 1850–2000*. New Delhi: Oxford University Press, 2014.

Sheth, D.L., 'Caste and Class: Social Reality and Political Representation'. In Pai Panadiker, V.A. & Nandy, Ashis Nandy. *Contemporary India*. New Delhi: Tata McGraw-Hill Publishing, 1999.

Siddiqui, Md Zakaria and Ronald Donato. 'Overweight and Obesity in India: Policy Issues from an Exploratory Multi-level Analysis.' *Health Policy and Planning*, 31, no. 5 (2016): 582–91.

Singh, Ajit Kumar. 'Why Jat Reservations?' *Economic & Political Weekly*, 46, no. 17 (2011): 20–22.

Singh, Malvika. *Perpetual City. A Short Biography of Delhi*. New Delhi: Aleph, 2013.

Sinha, Mrinalini. 'Giving Masculinity a History: Some Contributions from the Historiography of Colonial India.' *Gender & History*, 11, no. 3 (1999): 445–60.

Sitapati, Vinay. 'What Anna Hazare's Movement and India's New Middle Classes Say about Each Other.' *Economic & Political Weekly*, 46, no. 30 (2011): 39–44.

Spaaji, Ramón. 'Sport and Social Mobility: Untangling the Relationship.' In *Sport and Social Mobility: Crossing Boundaries*, pp. 16–40. New York: Routledge, 2011.

Smith, Aaron C.T. and Bob Stewart. 'Body Perceptions and Health Behaviors in an Online Bodybuilding Community.' *Qualitative Health Research*, 22, no. 7 (2012): 971–85.

Solomon, Harris. 'Unreliable Eating: Patterns of Food Adulteration in Urban India.' *Biosocieties*, 10, no. 2 (2015): 177–93.

Sreekumar, T.T. 'The Transnational Politics of the Techno-Class in Bangalore.' In *A Companion to Diaspora and Transnationalism*, edited by Ato Quayson and Girish Daswani, 539–55. Chichester, West Sussex: Wiley Blackwell, 2013.

Sridharan, E. 'The Growth and Sectoral Composition of India's Middle Class: Its Impact on the Politics of Economic Liberalization.' *India Review*, 3, no. 4 (2004): 405–28.

Srivastava, Sanjay. 'Fragmentary Pleasures: Masculinity, Urban Spaces, and Commodity Politics in Delhi.' *Journal of the Royal Anthropological Institute*, 16, no. 4 (2010): 835–52.

Srivastava, Sanjay. *Entangled Urbanism. Slum, Gated Community and Shopping Mall in Delhi and Gurgaon.* New Delhi: Oxford University Press, 2015.

Stallmeyer, John C. *Building Bangalore. Architecture and Urban Transformation in India's Silicon Valley.* London and New York: Routledge, 2013.

Stokvis, Ruud. 'The Emancipation of Bodybuilding.' *Sport in Society: Cultures, Commerce, Media, Politics*, 9, no. 3 (2006): 463–79.

Subrahmanyam, V.V. 'K. Venkatesan is Searching for a Decent Sponsorship to Take Part in Competitions.' *The Hindu*, 22 October 2017. Tamilnadu State Level Bodybuilding Competition. 'Steelman II: Tamil Nadu—2017 Award.' Ticket, 28 January 2017.

Strathern, Andrew J. *Body Thoughts*. Ann Arbor: University of Michigan Press, 1996.

Stutley, Margaret and James Stutley. *A Dictionary of Hinduism*. London: Harper & Row, 1977.

Telang, Vrushali. *Can't Die for Size Zero*. New Delhi: Rupa Publications, 2010.

Tripathi, Amarnath and Shraddha Srivastava. 'Interstate Migration and Changing Food Preferences in India.' *Ecology of Food and Nutrition*, 50, no. 5 (2011): 410–28.

Turner, Bryan S. 'Body.' *Theory, Culture & Society*, 23, no. 2-3, (2006): 223–36.

Valiani, Arafaat A. 'Physical Training, Ethical Discipline, and Creative Violence: Zones of Self-Mastery in the Hindu Nationalist Movement.' *Cultural Anthropology*, 25, no. 1 (2010): 73–99.

Van Wessel, Margit. 'Talking about Consumption: How an Indian Middle Class Dissociates from Middle-Class Life.' *Cultural Dynamics*, 16, no. 1 (2004): 93–116.

Vasudev, Shefalee. 'The New Second Sex. Exploited, Underpaid, Underemployed, and Still Dreaming, the Agony of the Indian Male Model.' *Open*, 24 November 2017. http:// www.openthemagazine. com/article/cover-stor y/the-new- second-sex.

Voelcker, Verena Michael Sticherling, Jürgen Bauerschmitz. 'Severe Ulcerated 'Bodybuilding Acne' caused by Anabolic Steroid Use and Exacerbated by Isotretinoin.' *International Wound Journal*, 7, no. 3 (2010): 199–201.

Vohra, Paromita. 'Automatic Bodies.' *The Indian Quarterly*, Oct–Dec 2018.

Wacquant, Loïc. 'Whores, Slaves and Stallions: Languages of Exploitation and Accommodation among Boxers.' *Body & Society*, 7, no. 2-3 (2001): 181–94.

Walkerdine, Valerie. 'Biopegogies and Beyond.' In *Biopolitics and the 'Obesity Epidemic': Governing Bodies*, edited by Jan Wright and Valerie Harwood, 199–207. New York & London: Routledge, 2009.

Waskul, Dennis D. and Phillip Vannini. 'Introduction: The Body in Symbolic Interaction.' In *Body/Embodiment: Symbolic Interaction and the Sociology of the Body*, edited by Dennis Waskul and Phillip Vannini, 1–18. England: Ashgate, 2006.

Watt, Carey A. 'Cultural Exchange, Appropriation and Physical Culture: Strongman Eugen Sandow in Colonial India, 1904–1905.' *The International Journal of the History of Sport*, 33, no. 16 (2016): 1921–42.

Wedemeyer, Bernd. 'Body-building or Man in the Making: Aspects of the German Bodybuilding Movement in the Kaiserreich and

Weimar Republic.' *The International Journal of the History of Sport*, 11, no. 3 (1994): 472–84.

Weigers, Yvonne. 'Male Bodybuilding: The Social Construction of a Masculine Identity.' *Journal of Popular Culture*, 32, no. 2 (1998): 147–61.

Williams, Robert J. and Lina A. Ricciardelli. 'Social Media and Body Image Concerns: Further Considerations and Broader Perspectives.' *Sex Roles*, 71 (2014): 389–92.

Wright, Jan. 'Biopower, Biopedagogies and the Obesity Epidemic.' In *Biopolitics and the 'Obesity Epidemic': Governing Bodies*, edited by Jan Wright and Valerie Harwood, 1–14. New York & London: Routledge, 2009.

Yajnik, C.S. 'Symposium on 'Adipose Tissue Development and the Programming of Adult Obesity'—Obesity Epidemic in India: Intrauterine Origins?' *Proceedings of the Nutrition Society*, 63 (2004): 387–96.

# ACKNOWLEDGEMENTS

## Anonymity and Research-Friendships

Research for this book was conducted on-and-off over a ten-year period. During this time, I visited India numerous times. However, the bulk of the interviews and data gathering took place during nine months in Delhi (2013–14) and three in Chennai (2015). My Delhi-based fieldwork was made possible as part of a fellowship with the then newly established Nalanda University; while my stay in Chennai was facilitated through funding by the Asia Research Institute of the National University of Singapore. Many of the trainers and bodybuilders I met and interviewed during these phases became friends which allowed me to follow their lives over a much longer period. They were always well-aware of my intentions to write a book about the topic and would sometimes indicate for certain aspects or happenings not to be mentioned. I would like to thank all trainers, bodybuilders and others involved in the fitness industry for sharing their life stories, opinions and insights with me. Except for those informants whose opinions and life-course trajectories are already part of the public domain, all names in this book have been anonymised. I know this will disappoint some informants who were keen on having their real names featured in the book. However, this was not possible due to the following reason: even if informants were fully informed about how their stories were to be treated in this book, they were not aware of the broader context in which their narratives and life-course histories are discussed. If we consider a chapter as a space of characters brought together to make a particular argument, these characters themselves are not necessarily aware that they will occupy and share this space in such a manner. I am reminded of an instance some years ago when I was invited on stage at a bodybuilding competition to garland some of the winners. The chief moderator of the organising federation introduced me as 'Michael, a researcher who has come to write about us bodybuilders!' He was mightily pleased that I had come to tell 'their' stories and how well they were doing. With roughly 5,000 people in the audience and some 150 competing bodybuilders about to take the stage, he encouraged me to speak a few words of encouragement. I found that my research was often interpreted as having the potential to set the record straight, and that my writing would highlight the struggles Indian bodybuilders face in the absence of official governmental support. While it's my sincere hope that the situation of lack of support changes in the future, I did not embark on this research project with this specific objective in mind. Considering the nature of academic research, it was not always easy to get this across.

## A Word of Thanks

I owe a debt of gratitude to my agent Kanishka Gupta who for not altogether clear reasons believed in this book from the start. At Context, I thank the wonderful Ajitha for her amazing editing, and Karthika for her enthusiasm in taking on this book. It's presses like Context that allow authors like myself to unshackle ourselves from academic constraints and to seek a wider audience for the research we have conducted.

I would like to thank Nalanda University's former vice-chancellor, the formidable Gopa Sabharwal, and her right-hand, the inspiring Anjana Sharma, for their unrelenting support. At the Asia Research Institute of the National University of Singapore, I am particularly grateful to Jonathan Rigg, the institute's director, and Brenda Yeoh, one of the institute's leading academics for providing a deeply inspiring work environment. I would also like to acknowledge the Institute for Social and Economic Change in Bangalore, for kindly hosting part of the research, and Sujata Patel for facilitating important contacts there.

Over the years, the research has benefitted from countless conversations, discussions and suggestions from academic colleagues, journalists and friends. First of all, I would like to express my deep appreciation for Itty Abraham's encouragement to turn the material on hand into a book. He saw 'a book' long before I had the courage to admit that maybe I did so too. I would also like to mention my dear friend and colleague Michelle Miller here. Co-confidante and researcher extraordinaire herself, it was our long-term conversations about research and related predicaments that inspired and gave me the courage to carry on. Ronojoy Sen, who was writing his unmatched *A History of Sports in India* (2015) when we were at the same institute, and Joseph Alter, who joined Yale-Nus as a visiting professor of anthropology at the same time, should not be omitted here either. Sen's encouragement and Alter's enthusiasm for this book, as well as his own profound work in the field of Indian masculinities, were crucial to the project at large.

In an earlier phase, the project benefitted immensely from input from a number of colleagues and friends. Caroline Osella was one of the first to believe that this was a project that begged further investigation. Similarly, Amsterdam-based Niko Besnier, Jeroen de Kloet, Giselinde Kuipers, Annemarie Mol, Mattijs van de Port, Rachel Spronk, Sylvia Tidey and Peter van der Veer all provided important input to fine-tune its focus. In the years to come, I would receive excellent advice, guidance and suggestions from Sunil Amrith, Baptist Coelho, Assa Doron, Roos Gerritsen, Knut Axel Jacobsen, Mathangi Krishnamurthy, Ritty Lukose, Kama Maclean, Shekhar Krishnan, Omita Goyal, Chris McMorran, Ursula Rao, Parmesh Shahani, Atreyee Sen, Sanjay Srivastava, Luisa Steur, Meredith Weiss and many others.

However, none of the research would have been made possible without a number of exceptionally brilliant friends. From the first time we met, film-maker and author Ashish Sawhny became a close friend and courteously opened his Bandra West apartment for my regular visits to Mumbai. Over time, I also collaborated with NTU scholar and anthropologist Julien Cayla, which led to an insightful comparison between fitness trainers and coffee baristas as new service professionals in urban India. Sudeep Sen—at whose house I stayed with while in Delhi in 2013–14—proved to be invaluable for the way the project took shape. In later years, staying with John Conolly and Atanu Majindar at their GK-I apartment similarly offered the opportunity to reacquaint with old friends while also discussing research findings at length. It often goes unsaid but it is undeniable that long-term ethnographic fieldwork, such as lies at the heart of this book, depends on such kindness. Similarly,

Delhi-friends Mishty Varma (and her delightfully barefooted husband Suchetha), as well as Jaya Bhattacharji Rose, Shovon Choudury and Vikram Chauhan all shared important insights and offered important suggestions over the years.

Conversations in 'the South' similarly helped the book take shape. I am deeply grateful of Dirk Gastman for his uncanny habit of revealing rather inherent truths about India, a country which he as a 'Belgian man' has now called home for forty years. Surendran and Rajesh Calambakam have always cheerfully opened their Bangalore home to me and provided me with invaluable insight into the way the city operates. Akash Kapur, Tishani Doshi and Carlo Pizzati's encouragement was also of influence here, reminding me of the possibilities of the material on hand, and what could be accomplished by it. Finally, there is Chitra Venkataramani, Meenakshi Shedde, Arshia Sattar and Rupleena Bose who over the years not only remained important sources of information, but also suggested intriguing new ways of approaching the material.

This book is dedicated to my partner, friend for life and love of my life, Rithesh Calambakam. I can only wish that every researcher has a partner like this; one who is unwavering in his opinion of *this* being a silly hobby, at most something that keeps me off the street and at worst something that is pretentious and self-important. It keeps me sane and healthy. There is simply no person I love more.

# INDEX

narrative about, 4
new and old India, dichotomy between, 38
new and shining, 8
newness discourse of, 37
new India,
    construction of, 38
    disillusionment with, 140
    idea of, 37, 270n58
    transformation of, 3, 4, 37–41, 43
Indian masculinities, 151, 152
Indians, belittling of, 105
international bodybuilding, 163
intimacy, 238–41
IT professionals, family trajectories of, 40
Iyer, K.V., 232

Jain, Rimjhim, 144
Jat agitation, 183
Jats, 173
Jaura, Samir, 30
Jayaraman, Gayatri, 139–40
Jodhka, Surinder S., 9
joriclub swinging, 236, 283n223
Joshi, Sanjay, 6

Kapoor, Anand, 158–59
Kapoor, Arjun, 229
Kapur, Akash, 141
Karan, 147–48
Kesavan, Mukul, 269n53
Khamkar, Suhas, 107
Khan, Aamir, 2
Khan, Salman, 1, 34
Khan, Shah Rukh, 2, 33
Kimmel, Michael, 150
kirana shops, 275n118
Klein, Alan M., 97, 233

Kolkata, 142
Kollywood, 268n46

Lacan, Jacques, 237
Landholdings, subdivision of, 184
life coaching, 82
life, quality of, 3

Macaulay, Lord T.B., 5
Mainardi, Robert, 232
male bodily ideals, globalisation of, 29
male body, sexual capital of, 227–31
male fashion industry, exploitation of, 224–25
male model, 208, 212, 223, 225, 227
Man of Madras, 209
Manikrao, Rajratan, 106
*Marichika*, 223–24
marriage, 270n53
masculine strength and athleticism, 1
masculinity,
    crisis of, 164
    manly virtues, 151
    performance of, 153
    social norms of, 150
Mawdsley, Emma, 7
*Memento*, 2
*Men's Health*, 37, 99–100
    ceasing of publication, 268n47
    launch of Indian edition of, 2, 35, 36
middle class, 13–15
    colonial middle class in north India, 6
    demands of, 10
    growth of, 3
    new middle class, behaviour of, 170

www.ingramcontent.com/pod-product-compliance
Lightning Source LLC
Chambersburg PA
CBHW070055030426
42335CB00016B/1895

* 9 7 8 9 3 9 5 0 7 3 6 2 2 *